QUALITY
HOSPICE
CARE

QUALITY HOSPICE CARE

Administration, Organization, and Models

Alice McDonnell, Dr. P.H.

Foreword by
Jack Zimmerman, M.D.

(NHP) **NATIONAL HEALTH PUBLISHING**
A Division of RYND COMMUNICATIONS

Printed in the United States of America
First Printing
ISBN: 0-932500-36-6
LC: 85-62898

CONTENTS

PART II

HOSPICE MODELS OF CARE

Foreword

Among the remarkable features of hospice care is its adaptability to a wide spectrum of needs and capabilities. The increasing application of hospice principles over the last several years has raised a number of questions and issues, such as the effectiveness of hospice care, as well as the strengths of each type of hospice care.

Forthrightly and in considerable detail, this book addresses two critical and complex issues in hospice today; namely, quality of care and the relative merits of various organizational approaches.

Each of us involved in providing comfort to the dying must achieve high quality care. Regardless of the hospice design, quality of care assurance must be the common denominator. Thus, although difficult, quality must be measured and evaluated concurrently. Society will inevitably supplement these internal controls by imposing some type of external control. In any case, without combining both skillful management *and* compassion, hospice programs will surely fail.

Systematic classification of hospice programs is likewise essential in comparing the various types of hospice organization, but such categorization is fraught with a number of problems. This book eases the confusion by explaining the most common groupings in hospice care. These include hospital, home care, freestanding, community, and skilled nursing. As the hospice movement grows, additional classifications or subgroupings will arise, adding to the difficulties in providing effective management. Indeed, there are some hospice programs today which don't fit well into any category. Fundamental approaches to hospice management, however, can be applied to any hospice design.

The importance of continuity in hospice care cannot be minimized. Fragmentation has interfered greatly with the treatment of the terminally ill. One particularly troublesome form of fragmentation is the loss of continuity as the patient moves between sites of care: hospital, intermediate care facility, home. Of enormous value to patient and family is the consistent availability of hospice practices as the appropriate care setting changes.

As one confronts these matters of quality of care and comparison of hospice models, some interlocking issues arise. First, several points regarding finances are important. Cost and reimbursement are not the same; understanding the distinction can be of critical importance to all hospice workers. Furthermore, whereas most of us who have been involved in the initiation of hospice programs see them as providing improved quality of care in a cost-effective manner, public policy may now be looking at hospice *primarily* as an instrument of cost containment. In addition, reimbursement will undoubtedly be used as a measure to control quality. This is not only inevitable, but for the most part commendable. The threat which it poses to innovation, however, must be dealt with realistically. We must also deal with the issue of how many hospices are needed; the balance between needs and numbers is likely to affect both quality and cost.

As Dr. McDonnell stresses throughout this book, the hospice concept should tie into general medical care. The problems which occur in the management of the terminally ill are neither unique to our time and technology, nor unique to the dying. Severe illness and incapacity and approaching death have always been threatening and overwhelming. In a sense, the care of the terminally ill mirrors all of medical care. If indifference and lack of respect for personal autonomy create impediments to the proper care of the dying, they do also for those who will get well. Expanding application of hospice philosophy offers an opportunity for a favorable impact on all of medical care. For example, those of us in medicine may need to re-learn that our *first* step in dealing with a patient is not necessarily to take a history and do a physical examination, but rather to make him comfortable.

Conversely, hospice care suffers when it stands in isolation from the remainder of medicine. There is no question that some aggressive measures commonly associated with curative treatment can be utilized effectively in palliation. For the patient with cancer, this may be anti-tumor therapy such as radiation or the pinning of a painful pathologic fracture to provide comfort. The point is that hospice and the remainder of medical care must not only co-exist, but cooperate.

Another valuable feature of this book is its emphasis on the importance of research in hospice care. There are many avenues of investigation which must be followed. The provision of optimal quality of life is one of the overriding objectives of hospice care. If we are to determine the relative merits of different techniques, we must be able to measure, in some fashion, the quality of life. Whereas quantity is relatively easy to assess, quality poses immense difficulties. For example, there is the matter of value differences: what is desirable to one individual may be intolerable to another. Possibly, we will be able to measure *specific qualities* rather than the *overall quality* of life.

The growth and development of hospice philosophy, principles, and practice over recent years has been encouraging, perhaps even thrilling. The success of hospice thus far, however, does not guarantee its future, but rather raises more questions.

Excellence in care of the terminally ill will be a function of the emphasis placed upon quality assurance. The optimal design for a particular hospice program must be based upon specific needs and capabilities in the setting in which the program is developing. This book should help in making rational decisions with respect to these matters.

J. M. Zimmerman, M.D.

Preface

A major problem for individuals with a life-threatening illness is lack of sensitivity by health care professionals who provide care. Care of the terminally ill patient represents a significant gap in our health care system. At present the hospice movement is rapidly increasing without the benefit of empirical data or research to estimate the best organizational format conducive to the needs of hospice patients and their families. According to the Joint Commission for Accreditation of Hospitals (JCAH), in 1981 there were 440 operational programs, whereas in May 1984 JCAH reported an estimated 1,500.

A variety of structurally distinct models of hospice programs have emerged. Five major hospice models in the United States are the hospital-based, home care-based, freestanding, community-based, and skilled nursing models. The growth of hospices throughout the United States poses potential questions for health policymakers regarding the most appropriate structural arrangement, staffing patterns, reimbursement mechanisms, quality controls, and integration into the health care system.

Early in my nursing career I made a professional commitment to the patient with incurable disease. The hospice concept has allowed me to pursue that commitment on several levels and in various ways. This book has evolved from both my professional experiences in a hospice program as a clinician, administrator, and educator, and through personal experiences from the loss of loved ones. In addition, much of the information is based on my educational background: I conducted an exploratory research project, analyzing the basic models to determine the extent of their effectiveness in meeting selected criteria related to both quality and cost. In that no one organizational model for hospice care has emerged, it is necessary for health service administrators to know the benefits and detriments of the various models which have emerged. Since a common philosophy and purpose characterizes the hospice movement, it is important for health care providers to identify if and how the elements of hospice care are successfully transferred and implemented into the specific models. Although the hospice concept is neither problem-free nor issue-free, the philosophical base of the program is a humane, holistic approach to patient/family care that has gained support among many elements of society.

One of the purposes of this book is to emphasize the importance of professional management in order to provide quality care.

This book is designed not just for hospice administrators but also for many other individuals and professionals involved with administration of hospitals, nursing homes, home care agencies, public health departments, community agencies, and allied health institutions. It has also been written for practicing physicians, nurses, social workers, therapists (physical, speech, occupational, respiratory), nutritionists, pharmacists, spiritual counselors, and volunteers as well as board members of hospices, hospitals, skilled and intermediate care facilities, and voluntary agencies.

The book is useful as a text for management-oriented courses in graduate and undergraduate programs in hospital and health care administration and health planning, and in schools of allied health, dentistry, medicine, nursing, public health, business, and social work. The range of material is organized as a useful reference source for nonadministrative health professionals who are committed to the organization and delivery of quality hospice care. Rising expectations for the level and quality of hospice care have greatly increased and will continue to affect the demand for hospice services in communities. I have often received calls from leaders in other communities asking how to start a hospice program based on the multifaceted aspects of health care. It is my hope that this volume will answer basic questions as well as address comprehensive issues. It is, therefore, also intended for health care planners, policymakers, researchers, and consultants. For practitioners, this handbook offers practical application of the hospice concept within the health care delivery system. It also provides an overview for students in related disciplines such as health economics and medical sociology.

I hope that the insight I offer into the dynamics of hospice care will spur the development of new hospice programs. For additional resource material, please refer to the bibliography and "For Further Reading," beginning on p. 287.

Acknowledgements

The planning, preparation, and writing of this book has required the support of many people in many ways. As an administrator, professor, and clinician, I have been influenced by students, staff, board and committee members, colleagues, and other professionals who work closely with me from day to day and who have been in close contact with terminally ill people. Much of the book's content is derived from my own experiences as a hospice nurse and administrator.

I am grateful to my doctoral committee for their inspiration and encouragement. To Dr. Melanie Dreher, Chairperson, Dr. Lois Grau, Dr. Lowell Bellin, and Dr. Ruth Bennett, I shall always be indebted for their personal instruction. To Sonja Johansen, M.P.A., Ph.D. in biostatistics from Columbia University, a special thanks for her guidance in data compilation and analysis.

To the administrators, board, and staff of the sites used for the initial research, I give special appreciation and credit for their time and assistance. And to my typist, Linda Kellett, for her tireless assistance, I am deeply grateful.

A very special thanks goes to our patients and their families who have played a central role. It is from them I have learned the most about hospice care.

Finally, my children deserve kudos for their continuous patience and understanding.

Introduction

HOSPICE CARE: AN OVERVIEW

Hospice care for terminally ill patients and their families is a relatively new concept in the United States. As a specialized program of care, hospice is characterized ideally by comprehensive, continuous twenty-four hour services by an interdisciplinary team of professionals, nonprofessionals, and volunteers with central administration and physician direction for palliative and supportive care of the dying and their families. The interdisciplinary team--comprised of physicians (oncologists, primary care physicians, psychiatrists), professional nurses, medical social workers, therapists (physical, speech, occupational), home health aides, social work assistants, nutritionists, pharmacists, clergy, and volunteers--supervises and coordinates the plan of care for each individual patient and family. Hospice is geared to those with incurable illnesses for whom the terminal phase is of a known and relatively short duration.

The hospice concept promotes home care so that patients can maintain their lifestyle. Unlike the traditional curative hospital care, hospice care treats the symptoms rather than the disease. Hospice is concerned with emotional, spiritual, social, and economic stresses as well as physical aspects of pain. Finally, hospice programs provide bereavement counseling, seeking to assure the patient and families that they will not be abandoned and helping the survivors deal with the impact of death.

Hospice philosophy combines medical knowledge with reverence for life; it recognizes the spiritual needs that allow the patient and family to live as fully and comfortably as possible with meaning and dignity. Hospice recognizes dying as a normal process whether or not it is the result of disease. In order to provide continuity and flexibility, hospice services are provided on an inpatient, home care, and outpatient basis.

While there is no dearth of information about the type of care hospices should provide, various organizational strategies are being initiated with limited knowledge of their relative merits and suitability.

At the present time there is limited baseline data for comparison of hospices with conventional services. Both on a state and national level, basic hospice population characteristics are not available. The limitation on the quantity and quality of data available is surprising in light of the number of programs in existence and the multitude of governmental studies undertaken. Programs throughout the United States have not been in existence long enough to have generated sufficient quantitative data. Hospice programs are rarely in a position to fund extensive follow-up and analysis from their own resources. Budgetary constraints make it unlikely that anything but cursory information is gathered since compilation and analysis of the resulting information is beyond the limits of agency resources. Extensive background information, for example, or precisely-gathered case histories have no utility to the staff of most agencies. Compounding this situation is the fact that most grants for service to hospice patients emphasize the service rather than the research aspects of the program. Data deficiencies can also be explained by a concern on the part of hospice programs for maintaining the privacy of patients and their families to the maximum extent possible. While this serves to protect privacy, it is difficult for researchers to obtain accurate profiles of patient/family groups even when the data are aggregated. The execution of a precise research design is elusive in such circumstances. Therefore, it is intended that this book will contribute to the much-needed body of data pertaining to hospice.

MODELS OF HOSPICE CARE: A CONCERN FOR QUALITY

For the purposes of this book, quality of care is defined as the provision of the best possible array of needed hospice services for each patient and family. To operationalize this concept, research was based upon selected criteria from professional experiences and National Hospice Organization (NHO) standards. Levels of quality are ascertained by the presence or absence of identified basic hospice characteristics in the varied models of care: hospital-based, home care-based, freestanding, community-based, and skilled-nursing. These basic hospice characteristics also provide guidelines for efficient care to control costs yet provide a quality program.

The differences and similarities in the hospice models are discussed as to their formal and informal structure, functions, staffing patterns, resources available, funding sources, the quality of care they provide, and the effects of this care on the patient, family, and hospice staff. The success of hospice proponents in negotiating funding for capital expenses and reimbursement is affected by their ability to demonstrate the cost-saving potential of hospice.

This book is intended for hospice proponents as a comparison and analysis of hospice models with regard to the quality, cost, range of services they provide, and the extent to which their services are congruent with the basic characteristics of hospice programs. Hospices differ in their institutional location, organizational structure, and reimbursement mechanisms. Each model is described according to structural factors, relationship with the parent institution, table of organization, composition and education of personnel, patient charges and source of funding reimbursement, size and nature of the caseload, mechanism for provision of services, and manner in which services are provided. These factors are related first to patient/family satisfaction and, second, to the kind and amount of services provided to patients and families. The assessments of the varied hospice models articulate the relationship between quality, cost, and the organizational model in order to explain advantages and disadvantages to each specific model. Differences and similarities are explained, although this material is not intended to identify one model as the final word in hospice care. It is the responsibility of administrators to explore the potential of various models for providing services to the dying and their families. In addition, this book clarifies the major issues related to hospice administration. The intent is to provide insight into the dynamics of hospice care for use in the development of hospice programs. Hospice programs in the United States are highly individualized; each adapts to the special needs and resources of its own community. Since several organizational models for hospice care have emerged, it is important to know the advantages and disadvantages of those models by analyzing organizational structure, administrative practices, staffing patterns, and provision of care in each model. Since a common philosophy and purpose characterizes the hospice movement, it is important to identify if and how the goals of hospice care are successfully transferred and implemented into the specific models.

The literature on hospice care is concerned mainly with demonstrating the value of hospice compared with traditional methods of caring for the terminally ill. Some of the literature shows concern with quality and some authors are concerned with cost. Very little has been written comparing the various models of hospice with regard to these issues. Not only have questions not been answered regarding the relative merits of hospice care but they have not been asked.

Somers (1972) identifies five major themes that, to a large extent, set the stage for the development of various hospice models in our society:

1. The lifestyle of the consumer and problems of health education.

2. Availability of twenty-four-hour comprehensive care to overcome fragmentation and stress on acute inpatient care. More care should be rendered outside the hospital in less expensive settings, preferably at home, reducing costs and providing comprehensive care.

3. Rationalization of the delivery system. Comprehensive care must be made available to the entire population at the point of actual delivery, and payment for the services must be assured.

4. Redefinition of professional roles to assure personalized care.

5. Free-choice consumer responsibility and quality control. People have the right to determine the settings in which they

live and die and should not be denied appropriate health care if they choose to die at home.

The concept of hospice is, then, a caring rather than curing system, with services provided by a comprehensive team of practitioners. Care is offered to patient and family in a choice of environments, but especially in the home.

Hospice is not only a response to the existing status of health care but it stimulates to the system, to respond to changing societal values that emphasize the human being, free choice, and consumer awareness. Hospice is, therefore, the incentive for change as well as the outgrowth of societal change.

Hospice units within hospitals have provided evidence that when staff provides personalized care to hospice patients, improved patient care is the result. Some physicians have learned the value of the house calls made in conjunction with the care of hospice patients. Others have learned new skills in pain control and palliative care.

Hospice may be a home care program, a freestanding institution, a separate hospital department, or an interdisciplinary team that moves within a general hospital to wherever the patients may be located within the facility. A hospice program may offer outpatient services or day care; it may offer the home care in conjunction with the institutional settings; or it might combine variations of these models. The question of which model is the best for terminally ill patients is the focus for this book. Thus, hospice care can be given in a variety of ways and in various settings and under different kinds of auspices.

Due to regional differences, demographics, economics, methods of funding, staffing, and so on, different hospice models are operating in the United States. In some instances, the hospice movement is still largely experimental and in a state of flux, which naturally requires experimentation and adaptation to varied and changing circumstances. Widespread national initiatives are still in progress to (1) develop and coordinate systematic procedures, (2) study the solution of problems, funding, recruiting, and training of volunteers, and (3) attempt through education to overcome certain traditionally-entrenched cultural dogma and standards of the medical profession, hospitals, and administrators that have prevailed for years.

According to hospice standards, each model should be autonomous by having a specific hospice program and separate guidelines with a centrally administered program of coordinated inpatient and outpatient services in order to provide optimal utilization of services and resources. Ideally, the patient and family constitute the primary unit of care in conjunction with interdisciplinary hospice care team services provided by staff and volunteers with counseling and supportive services continued throughout the period of bereavement. There are variations within hospital-based and skilled nursing-based programs according to the individual organizational structure. The hospice may be comprised of a specific number of beds within a distinct unit or hospice beds may be integrated within the total hospital and skilled nursing setting served by a floating hospice team. The ideal hospice environment should contain such elements of the home environment as flowers, paintings, comfortable lounge chairs, libraries, sitting rooms, pets, and kitchen facilities. Children should be permitted in the hospice. Overnight accommodations for family and unlimited visiting hours are necessary in order to create a psychologically comfortable atmosphere conducive to the welfare of the patient. In contrast to a freestanding facility, hospital-based services are incorporated into an already existing facility; a unit is usually remodeled for this specific purpose. It functions as a part of the hospital but has its own staff, a hospice team especially trained to care for the dying and their families and who is paid by the hospital. Special units of this kind are usually exempted from some of the more stringent regulations of the hospital; for example, hospice patients are allowed to receive an unlimited number of visitors of any age around the clock. At the present time, the cost of hospice care in the hospital to the patient/family is determined by hospital financial policies.

The home care model uses either an existing traditional visiting nurse association or provides care in conjunction with a separate hospice corporation, a community-based model, that has achieved status as a certified home health agency and functions as an independent, interdisciplinary unit which cooperates with other home health agencies in the area.

For hospice patients who require short-stay, day care, or overnight services, the freestanding unit is the basic model. This respite type care may provide temporary relief for family members who need a break from the exhausting care at home but who must continue working to provide an ongoing income for the family. The freestanding autonomous hospices exist separately from other facilities and are independent from them. Ideally, however, these separate units are a component of a total hospice program where there is coordination with home care and hospital-based services.

A review of the literature demonstrates a relationship between administrative strategy and quality of care. Quality of care is one of the major issues facing the health care industry. Mayers, Norby, and Watson (1977) state that high quality care does not happen by chance; it is the result of deliberative decision making and administrative practices. The organizational structure serves as an administrative control only to the extent of the effectiveness and efficiency of the structure in meeting the objectives of the organization, that is, quality of care. There can be inefficiencies within organizational structure which contribute to the upward cost spiral and decrease the quality and quantity of care received for the dollar. Social anthropologist William Caudill (1967) reports studies showing the interrelatedness of actions in an institution which influence patient behavior; he demonstrates how administrative actions have therapeutic consequences and how ordinary human relations affect the progress of the patient. The degree to which the staff is satisfied ultimately is related to quality of care. No matter how qualified and capable the practitioner is, the system must provide the opportunity for the provision of high quality care. The Joint Commission on Accreditation of Hospitals (JCAH) standards state that there shall be an organized program developed to improve patient care by objective analysis of such care and by the correction of identified problems through a written plan by administration.

Administrative models in health care institutions have been developed to provide quality of care at reasonable cost. However, this has not been done within hospice programs. Traditionally, the discussion has centered on varied staffing arrangements within organizational structure (such as primary nursing versus the team approach versus task orientation) and its effect on quality and types of services provided. This book focuses on the critical components in hospice organization and administration and how they affect quality hospice services (see Chapter 2). This book should provide the reader with a wealth of material for analysis and synthesis. We hope the information will be useful for the application of hospice principles in the implementation of hospice care services.

REFERENCES

Caudill, William. (1967). *The Psychiatric Hospital As A Small Society.* Cambridge, MA: Harvard University Press.

Mayers, Marlene G., Ronald B. Norby, and Annita B. Watson. (1977). *Quality Assurance for Patient Care.* New York: Appleton-Century-Crofts.

Somers, Ann. (1972). The Nation's Health: Issues for the Future. *The Annuals* 399:166-174.

PART I

HOSPICE ORGANIZATION

Chapter 1

The Evolution of the Hospice Movement

ORIGINS OF HOSPICE CARE

A history of the hospice movement clearly reveals that hospice care is not a new development, but rather a return to old values. Hospice is viewed as a humanistic approach to health care which emphasizes individuality among patients and a total needs assessment of the patient and family for comprehensive services. Some hospice techniques represent new applications of old knowledge. Changing attitudes toward health care delivery and toward the care of the dying have created a milieu favorable to the development of hospice programs. The hospice concept of care, which originated in Europe, has recently been gaining acceptance in the United States with support among all elements of society.

The word hospice originates from the Latin word for both host and guest. During the early Middle Ages, hospices in and around western European countries were places of rest for weary travelers. These hospices, which were run by monastic orders of the Christian sect, offered care for all who needed it, not only the dying. During the Crusades in the thirteenth century, when many pilgrims were traveling to and from the Holy Land, hospices served as places of rest and refreshment. Several small hospices were generally located between several large hospitals established in the arena of the Crusade's conflicts, the Middle East. These establishments were designed to care for wounded persons returning to various homelands in Europe. There, special attention, good food, and clean warm clothing were provided to those weary travelers who were ill and dying in a strange land, far from home (Stoddard, 1978). The caretakers of that period were imbued with a religious fervor that has rarely been duplicated in the last two centuries. (During the nineteenth century, the Irish Sisters of Charity established homes in Ireland, with what would have been then considered a skilled-nursing facility.) These places, unlike acute care hospitals, were small and quiet. Concomitantly, other hospices were being established in both England and France on a modest scale, creating the foundation for the modern British hospice system.

Two women played a major role in developing the hospice concept: Dr. Cicely Saunders of Great Britain and Dr. Elisabeth Kubler-Ross of the United States. Dr. Kubler-Ross, as an associate professor of psychiatry at the University of Chicago, first introduced the principles that are now encompassed in the philosophy of hospice. In the early 1960s, her well-publicized lectures on death and dying characterized the natural phenomenon of death (Guthrie, 1979). Where the terminally ill were concerned, she placed particular emphasis on providing complete pain control, sympathy, and care. Essentially, Dr. Kubler-Ross teaches the value of a positive acceptance of death rather than the denial that our society prefers. According to Dr. Kubler-Ross human beings have an inherent biological instinct for life, or a will to live, which insures survival of the species. Dr. Kubler-Ross (1975) writes:

> It will always be hard to die, but if we can learn to reintroduce death into our lives so that it comes not as a dreaded stranger but as an expected companion to our life, then we can learn to live our finiteness.

Dr. Kubler-Ross coined the phrase "dying with dignity." Control of pain, a prominent feature of hospice care, also helps the terminally ill patient live more fully until he or she dies. Dr. Kubler-Ross (1974) notes: "It is very difficult to maintain emotional equilibrium when you are in extreme pain."

Although Dr. Kubler-Ross espoused all the fundamental philosophy of the hospice concept, she did actively engage in establishing definite hospice organizations in this country. She was a staunch philosophical supporter of Dr. Cicely Saunders, who established the first hospice in Great Britain, and Kubler-Ross's theoretical work paved the way for the hospice movement to enter the United States. Dr. Kubler-Ross felt that most terminally ill patients prefer to die at home in familiar surroundings and in the presence of loved ones. However, she would compromise a home environment for an institutional surrounding which suggested a comfortable home atmosphere, devoid of tubes and electronic gadgetry. In the United States the focus of the hospice concept is primarily on a home care program. With the guidance of hospice personnel, some families are able to provide high quality care to their terminally ill members throughout the entire course of the illness. Patient and family know that the hospice is there when and if they need it.

The most visible aspect of the hospice to a community is likely to be the building and grounds. Some people might be inclined to regard hospice as a dismal "house of death" set apart from the community of the living. Actually, however, the hospice becomes part of the family and the community through its home care program. Emphasis is upon the total well-being of the terminally ill person--and the family--wherever they happen to be at the moment. Furthermore, the social and physical environment of the hospice is designed for active participation in life. Hospice is people-oriented and patient-centered.

Special concern for the dying is the latest development in what psychologist Robert Kastenbaum (1977) calls "the death-awareness movement." This movement represents a major effort to counter the effects of a very recent shift in the site and circumstances of dying. In 1900, two-thirds of Americans who died were under fifty years old, and most of them died in their own beds. Today, most

Americans are over sixty-five and confined to hospitals or nursing homes when they die. This removal of death from home to hospital greatly accelerated what French social historian Philippe Aries (1974) calls "a brutal revolution in traditional ideas and feelings."

At the extremes, Western attitudes toward death have ranged from those of the death cultists of the Black Plague to the romantic morbidity of Victorian poetry. But in Aries' authoritative outline of the past 2,000 years, early Western humans accepted death as his or her destiny--familiar, ordinary, and expected. The dying seemed to know when the end was near and placed great importance on preparing themselves. Death was a public ritual organized by the dying person in his or her bedchamber with neighbors, family, and priest attending.

From the Middle Ages onward, however, death and dying were subjected to subtle modifications. On the one hand, the dying developed a greater sense of personal identity so that death was no longer just a common destiny, but an individual experience. How one endured the trial of dying became the final test in determining how one would spend eternity. On the other hand, controls over the deathbed rituals gradually passed from the dying person to members of the family, who sought to ease the burden by avoiding references to the impending death. By the mid-nineteenth century, the postmortem rituals--funeral processions, the wearing of mourning clothes, and visits to the cemetery--had superseded the deathbed rituals. Although death was still public, dying had already become a relatively private affair.

By the mid-twentieth century, Aries observes, death was rapidly disappearing from public view in the industrialized Western nations. Today, techniques of modern medicine that prolong life also rob death of its personal and social significance. Through drugs and machines, the dying live on while death arrives in stages; neither the patient nor the physician can always tell when the final moment has come. Afterward, the denial of death sets limits to mourning; deep grief must be controlled and vented only in private. And the increasing popularity of cremation--it is now the dominant form of disposition in England-- confirms Aries' opinion that the once familiar face of death has become, in Western societies, something "shameful and forbidden."

Anne Munley (1983) describes her experiences in hospice settings in England and the United States which emphasize the importance of the philosophic and religious aspects of highly personalized terminal care. The literature as well as the author's experience confirms the significance of pastoral care on the quality of hospice service. The presence of a chaplain on a hospice team helps to articulate spiritual problems which otherwise would get only superficial treatment. A chaplain who knows medical language and the milieu of the hospital may be better able to help as part of a hospice team than the parish clergyman called in to deal with occasional problems.

Because of the reluctance of some cultures and religions to handle death and dying, the need for hospice arose with a goal to remove the stigma of death and the isolation that accompany the institutionalized way of dying. Hospice recalls the medieval concept of "the good death", where one ended one's life surrounded by family and friends, forgiving grievances and, in turn, being forgiven. Hospitals today do not provide an environment in which dying can be a positive experience.

According to Noyes and Clancy (1977), society is failing to meet the obligation it has to its dying members. Persons with terminal illnesses suffer isolation and neglect in hospitals, receive overzealous treatment by physicians, and are kept in ignorance of their situation by families and medical personnel. Evidence for these statements has come from observers of the medical care system and from dying patients themselves.

The now-fashionable dogma that the dying should accept their death turns out, however, upon reflection and experience, to be subject to serious reservations. For some individuals, accepting the imminence of death would be so out of character, so at variance with the pattern of their lives, so contrary to their repeated explicit desires, that one can only recoil at the occasional well-meaning effort to compel them to acknowledge their impending death "for their own good." Such an approach, smacking of the most audacious kind of paternalism, quite ignores the fact that acceptance may not be an appropriate coping mechanism for all individuals (Halper, 1979). Some patients, for instance, seem to prefer denial, and anecdotal evidence has not established this to be an inferior approach. For acceptance, after all, may strike the individual as fundamentally incompatible with hope, a stance universally praised both as a matter of human compassion and because of the statistical impossibility of predicting the outcome of specific cases. How can one be hopeful and accepting of one's own death at the same time? The answer, of course, is that many persons cannot. For some, attempts at acceptance undermine enclaves of hope; their resulting despair and desolation is not much relieved by reports that others have found acceptance agreeable. Therefore, the hospice program may not be appropriate for every terminal patient/family.

Nevertheless, the general philosophy of hospice has proved most successful. Dr. Cicely Saunders, the aggressive idealist who actually launched the hospice movement in her native Great Britain, established Saint Christopher's Hospice in Sydenham, England--the first functioning hospice institution. Dr. Saunders' field experience as a nurse combined with her qualities as a physician laid the foundation for a whole new concept of care for the terminally ill (Goldenberg, 1979). She set out to study symptom control scientifically and to acknowledge all the needs of the dying patient. Most of the hospice organizations which have been established since then have followed her principles of care. She was extremely successful and she inspired physicians, professional nurses, social workers, and volunteers internationally to function as members of a hospice team.

Located in a quiet middle-class suburb, Saint Christopher's is a well-known and highly regarded hospice often used as a model for emerging programs in the United States. The program at Saint Christopher's supports quality of life rather than extension of life beyond the patient's ability to endure living (Dunphy, 1979). The pain control theories developed by Dr. Saunders provide the basis for understanding the underlying concept of hospice care. Based on careful observation of the patient's needs, medication dosages are monitored and frequently adjusted to enable the hospice patient to spend his or her last days as alert, pain-free, and responsive to life as possible. Saint Christopher's also incorporates and stresses the multidisciplinary team approach. Headed by a physician who directs all activities, the hospice team regards the patient and family together as the unit of care. Hospice programs in the United States today emphasize team meetings, staff support systems, and continuing in-service education.

Sociologists, politicians, and clergy agree that the family is the "cement" that holds most societies together. However, many sociological, economic, and technological changes have altered this ideal. Earlier generations remember when the members of families who were seriously ill were cared for in their own home or in the homes of close extended family. This procedure was almost an unwritten social code for our society and was followed unless the home was unsuitable, in which case the patient regretably was hospitalized. Even then, upon discharge from the hospital, the home was the preferred setting for convalescence, attended with good family care and extended family participation. Hospitals were regarded as asylums for the "sick poor" or a retreat for "wealthy eccentrics" (Cunningham, 1979). A member from the average so-called respectable family customarily died at home surrounded by family and neighbors. The family doctor came and went. Occasionally, there was a nurse who came and stayed during those last days. The deceased family member was attended by an undertaker at home, and the remains rested in a casket in the "family parlor" until the interment day, two or three days later. The so-called wake or viewing was an accepted custom.

With the growth of the undertaking business in the last thirty-five years, these family customs have become increasingly depersonalized. Today, the deceased is whisked out of the home to the funeral parlor. The intimacy of family and neighbors has been further diluted by this development, and the age-old involvement of families has diminished.

Hospice care has shifted emphasis back to participation by the family. Patients and families are encouraged to share their feelings as they wish, to come to terms with the reality of the death, to plan the death rituals and the family's future, to proceed with "unfinished business," and to participate in anticipatory grief.

Hospice care in North America originated in 1975 with the opening of the Palliative Care Unit at the Royal Victoria Hospital in Montreal. During this time Hospice Incorporated of Connecticut was also being started with a home care program which further developed into a freestanding unit. Shortly thereafter, in 1977, the National Hospice Organization was formed in Washington, D.C. to provide information about hospice care and to establish and maintain standards of hospice care published in November 1981 by the National Hospice Organization. Stoddard (1978), Cohen (1979), and Spiegel (1983) vividly trace the historical development of hospice programs with excellent descriptions of hospice care. Below we will identify some of the more important influences surrounding the hospice concept in its evolution--cultural and social, economic, and political--which affect the varied organizational and administrative structures developed here in the United States.

CONCEPTUAL INFLUENCES

Cultural and Social Influences

Both historically and culturally, American people have found it difficult to cope with death, dying, and the terminally ill. The most typical response to learning of a terminal illness has been to recommend institutionalization. Efforts to prolong life have been made frequently through the use of highly sophisticated medical technology. Hospice programs have developed at least partly in response to our concern for the appropriate use of heroic measures in prolonging the lives of the terminally ill.

Perhaps the deepest reasons for our mismanagement of the death process in America stem from our heritage and our culture--what Kastenbaum and Aisenberg (1972) term our ''death system''--which constitutes all the thoughts, words, feelings, beliefs, and behavior that are related to death. All societies have developed at least one death system through which they come to terms with aspects of death in both personal and social ways. American society, however, faces a set of conditions concerning death that may be altering our cultural heritage in ways not yet understood. For the first time in human history, we no longer have an extremely limited life expectancy. We also now have increasingly large-scale control over natural forces. In addition, modern human beings have relatively little exposure to and a great deal of isolation from the sight of death. In the conventional hospital setting, the patient is frequently alone at the time of death. The body is transferred out as quickly as possible. However, in a hospice setting, the family is encouraged to be with the patient. If a family member is not available, staff stay with the patient. After the death, family may stay with the body, may touch it, and may pray together until they feel comfortable about leaving. Furthermore, the concept of individualism is now more developed than ever before in human history; modern humans now stand alone with considerably less support from clan, extended family, or city-state.

With the publication of Kubler-Ross's classic work, *On Death and Dying* (1969), a heightened awareness of this society's attitude toward those subjects and the problems faced by individuals whose lives are about to end have received increasing attention. Literature on this topic appears more frequently and ranges from accounts that deal with the personal experiences of dying persons to more technical reports of research in the improved control of pain in advanced malignancies. This trend represents only a beginning; American society basically remains a death-denying culture. For approximately two-thirds of those who die in this country each year, death does not take place at home but in institutions such as hospitals and nursing homes (Hendin, 1973). Many children in the United States grow to adulthood without having witnessed a death. The funeral custom of cosmetically making up those who have died so that they appear more lifelike helps perpetuate the widespread denial of death.

Although surveys reveal that most people would prefer to die at home, only a small percentage of patients are able to do so: hence, the impetus for the emphasis on hospice home care here in the United States. Hospitals, where many deaths occur, function primarily to cure acute illness or maximize recovery from chronic illness. The needs of a person in the terminal stage of an illness are not related to the performance of either of these functions, and a general hospital is therefore poorly equipped to meet them. The patient's psychological and emotional needs are viewed by the hospital's staff as subordinate to his or her physical needs. Staffing patterns involve repeated shifting of personnel; therefore, little time is available to staff for meeting a patient's emotional needs, and at times even physical needs must wait. Such organizational shortcomings are often compounded by the ambivalent attitudes of physicians and other hospital staff toward those who are dying. In a system that emphasizes cure at all costs, the dying represent a threat of failure, and they constantly remind staff members of their own mortality. Other problems encountered in hospitals by the terminally ill include the increasing bureaucratic restrictions on the length of hospital stay allowed a patient, a lack of comprehensive home care programs, inadequate support systems, fragmentation of care, depersonalization--the patient must fit the system and follow regulations--and emphasis on the disease process and technology.

Hospice is vastly different from conventionally practiced health care. The whole approach to care in hospice emphasizes that death is part of the life cycle. The dying person and his or her family are the core of concern for the hospice team. When the patient dies, the death itself changes the focus of attention from the deceased to the survivors. There may be both an outpouring of emotions as well as a sigh of relief that the suffering is over and the traumatic part of life is ended. Survivors are not at first exposed to the loss and the loneliness because of the focus on the many details, both financial and familial. Families and friends converge--where survivors are fortunate to have these concerned persons--but all at the same time. Then the visitors leave and the supports are reduced. It is at this time that hospice services reach out to the bereaved to complete the program of care.

In contemporary society, the mourners are urged to return to a state of normalcy as quickly as possible. Mourning, in most cases, actually lasts for at least a year and rushing its completion may prolong or intensify the entire process. It is for this reason that bereavement services should be available for that length of time. There is evidence to suggest that the traditional Irish wake or the Jewish shiva (culturally prescribed rituals following death) contribute to survivors' mental health. Grief is a necessary reaction to loss and is not a sign of weakness or self-indulgence. Funerals and other rituals concretize the reality of death and bring support to the bereaved person through the attention and concern of family and friends.

According to Williamson, Evans, and Munley (1982), by the 1960s, social factors influencing the family as an institution had created a shift in perception: care of the aged had begun to be viewed as a societal responsibility rather than a family responsibility. A number of factors contributed to the acceleration of this change in attitude: urbanization, industrialization, mandatory retirement, geographical mobility, an improved standard of living, higher levels of educational attainment by both men and women, smaller family size, breakdown in the family unit, increased numbers of women in the labor force, and a growing involvement of government in the affairs of the elderly. Changing role definitions of "wife" and "homemaker" increasingly influenced the lives of women who previously had been the primary caregivers for the aged and infirm. Although strong patterns of affective familial ties persist, physical care of the infirm elderly gradually moved out of the household into specialized institutions. Grandparents and elderly aunts and uncles incapable of maintaining a separate household or in need of custodial care could no longer be assured of a place in the home of younger relatives. In addition, there were numerous elderly persons who simply did not have any relatives on whom to rely. Some had outlived all family members; others lacked family ties because they had never married.

But changes in family form and functions were not the only factors leading to greater utilization of institutional care. The most striking event of the 1960s in terms of institutionalized care of the aged was the enactment of the Medicare and Medicaid programs in 1965. This legislation continued the politicalization of care of the elderly begun in the 1930s and publicly underscored the fact that a transferral of responsibility for the infirm aged from the family to the government had occurred. With the aging thus removed from the nuclear family, the succeeding generations become desensitized to death of the old. Hospitals isolated the ill. Therefore, because people rarely saw death, they could avoid it and in doing so, they feared it (Schoenberg and Carr, 1972). Dr. Balfour Mount (1974) described the vast changes in the North American way of life over the past fifty years:

> At the turn of the century we were an agrarian society. Birth, life and death were shared events. They occurred within the home environment and when Grandpa fell off the hay mow, he was laid out in the front parlor.
>
> Neighbors and grandchildren came to pay their last respects. We perhaps tend to romanticize the "death with dignity" that followed, but in any event, it was shared death. Death was seen as a part of life. It happened naturally, every day, and was seen in the context of nature with its cycles of life and death.

The high mortality rates associated with infancy, maternity and infections and other diseases helped to increase this sense of familiarity with death. Death could hardly be ignored.

Mount has noted other important recent developments:

- More than 70% of North Americans now die in institutions. Those suddenly taken seriously ill are frequently rushed to intensive care units of hospitals.

- Advances in modern medicine have enabled people to live longer--mortality rates have dropped. More and more diseases are curable; and even for those that are not, life can be considerably extended. To many physicians today, a death is a therapeutic failure.

- More people now die at an older age, and cardiovascular and malignant diseases now predominate as the major cause of death.

- As society has become more urban and more mobile, the natural life cycle is less obvious. Man is shielded from death.

- Belief in a religion and in the sanctity and ultimate significance of life has declined, and has frequently been replaced by a sense of meaninglessness.

- North American materialism and affluence have emphasized things and events rather than feelings and relationships.

- Modern mass communication and the entertainment medium have made mass deaths and individual murders so commonplace as to be unreal and unaffecting.

Glaser and Strauss (1965) in their seminal research in care of the dying look at the social consequences of dying for hospital staff as well as for patients and families. Because most people die in hospitals, these writers are concerned with the interaction between patients and hospital staff and argue for a more rational and compassionate response. They recognize that depriving the hospital staff member of the chance to hope for and work toward a complete recovery, results in a decrease in involvement and effort in patient care. An alternative emphasis, they point out, could be the redirection of nursing efforts toward "comfort care" which is more appropriate for the dying patient. Certainly hospice emphasizes this opportunity as there is always much more that can and should be done to relieve pain and other symptoms, such as distress, fear, and isolation. This time can be a period of growth for the patient, family, and staff.

Economic Influences

During the past ten years there has been critical public and governmental concern about the unrestrained spiraling of medical care costs in the United States. Dying persons routinely have received care that includes the use of expensive life-support systems and other extraordinary measures. The development of hospice programs has made a change in practice where some dying patients receive less expensive palliative care. Historically in the United States health services have tended to develop as a result of available health care dollars.

Hospices have been established through the creativity and commitment of volunteers. Such volunteers established the first hospice program in Connecticut and continue to be invaluable as direct caregivers, professional consultants, assistants in administration, members of the board of the directors, and advocates in the community. From the very beginning, professionals from the medical, nursing, social service, and religious disciplines worked with lay community leaders to establish hospice. They served on planning committees, spoke to community groups, and sought funds for hospice organizations.

Volunteers have participated in decisions on the details of procedure and policy development while rendering thousands of hours of patient and family service. Volunteers also participated in interdisciplinary team growth. Attendance at staff in-service education sessions and clinical conferences enable the core group to help with the integration of new volunteers. This enrichment of the curriculum for volunteers orientation and training continues in hospice program.

In August 1974, the director of volunteer services at the Connecticut Hospice, Inc. visited Saint Christopher's hospice and Saint Luke's Nursing Home in England to meet with volunteers and their supervisors for observation and consultation. It was evident that patients, families, and paid staff relied on quality volunteer service in roles that were uncommon in English general hospitals, sharing both caring tasks and caring relationships. The hospices had developed an environment where trust may grow between professionals and nonprofessionals; where patients, family members, volunteers, and staff join together to give and receive care; and where the inevitable blurring of roles reduces interdisciplinary tensions. Hospice personnel believe that such teamwork is necessary for the effective care of terminal patients.

To implement the hospice philosophy of care in this country, an organized structure for management of the volunteer program was needed. The provision of services by lay and professional volunteers requires written procedures to define training, reporting, supervision, and responsibility. The careful development of the volunteer program has provided a solid foundation for services that meet every discipline's standards, help to keep the cost of health care down, prevent duplication, and enhance the total package of care provided by hospice. It is important to point out that the conditions of participation for the hospice benefit under Medicare requires that five percent of the time spent giving patient care must be provided by a volunteer.

The success of hospice proponents in negotiating funding for capital expenses and reimbursement is affected by their ability to demonstrate hospice care's systems' cost-saving potential. A three-month study in 1979 of the patients in Church Hospital Hospice program revealed that the average per diem charge to the hospice patients was 44 percent less than the average per diem charge to the medical/surgical patients (Wehr, 1980). In an overbedded community, a hospice treating large numbers of patients might empty local hospital beds. In this situation, the hospital could be pressured into closing unused wings, or converting acute care beds for other uses, such as long-term care--perhaps with a hospice unit. Whether wings were converted to long-term care or a long-term/hospice combination, lower level staffing and cheaper allowable costs would result. Thus, a successful inpatient hospital-based hospice unit in a community might reduce the total number of acute care beds or convert excess beds to less expensive uses. Also hospice care in an underbedded or developing community could alleviate the need for construction of additional hospital beds. Patients who might otherwise have been hospitalized could be cared for outside the hospital with an approach that is proving to be less costly and more appropriate--hospice home care. At Royal Victoria Hospital, an analysis of home-care cases for a three-month period in 1976 showed that the average patient was saving eighty dollars a day, and the hospital was saving $130,900 for the period. This would free existing hospital beds for other patients, and help alleviate the community's original need for additional beds (Rossman, 1979). In addition, if it proved necessary to build some type of structure for hospice--involving relatively inexpensive facilities and equipment--the freestanding model would prove more economical than hospital construction. Current studies continue to reveal that hospice cost savings are substantial. The 1983 Ohio study found that hospice cost savings to third-party insurers were substantial representing a relative savings of approximately 40 percent by substituting less costly home care visits for more expensive hospital inpatient days (Brooks and Smyth-Staruch, 1983).

Political Influences

The government's first serious foray into hospice care began in October 1979 on the initiative of outgoing Health, Education, and Welfare--now Health and Human Services (HHS)--Secretary Joseph A. Califano, Jr. He spoke on October 5, 1978 to the National Hospice Organization (NHO), which had been formed in February 1977 to develop and promote standards of care, and gave a major boost to the fledgling but fast-growing hospice movement by announcing HEW's request for proposals for experimental funding of hospice programs. He established a Hospice Task Force consisting of representatives from various offices within HEW. The Task Force was directed by the Secretary to conduct research, gather data, and make recommendations to him regarding the potential role the federal government should play in support and development of hospice in the United States. At that time hospice also received endorsement from both ends of the congressional political spectrum when Senators Edward M. Kennedy (D--Massachusetts) and Bob Dole (R--Kansas) both called for increased federal funding of hospice programs (Hamilton and Reid, 1980). Califano, who reported spending a day in New Haven, Connecticut speaking to those involved with the New Haven Hospice, said he "went to New Haven with the idea that hospice was about dying. I came away realizing that hospice is something far more: it is about living, a way of living more fully and completely, embraced by human concern and support--up to, and through the end of life" (Califano, 1978).

At the request of Congress, the General Accounting Office (GAO) conducted an in-depth study of various organizations and agencies involved in hospice across the country. Much interest in the hospice movement had been generated by Congress but various legislators made it clear that more studies needed to be conducted before definitive legislation could be drafted.

In 1979, the Health Care Financing Administration (HCFA) made grant monies available to assist in the proposal of major health financing policy and program issues. HCFA's priority grant areas were as follows:

> Terminal Illness: studies of the costs and manner of the medical, social, and emotional problems posed by terminal illness; possible alternatives, such as home care or hospice care and their costs and effectiveness; examination of when the illness is or is not a medical issue; when should the Medicare or Medicaid program be responsible to pay costs "related" to the illness.

Senator Abraham Ribicoff joined Senators Kennedy and Dole in a bipartisan effort to call attention to this important issue. Their intent was described in the May 18, 1978 Congressional Record:

> We must all work together to provide for those in our society who are near death, an environment that recognizes (each of) them as an individual with dignity seeking only to spend (his) last days and hours peacefully in a manner of his choosing.

In the fall of 1979, twenty-six awards were made for demonstration projects throughout the United States through HCFA. At the same time the Hartford Foundation and the Robert Wood Johnson Foundation provided money to evaluate quality of care in these same demonstration projects. Finally, in 1982, legislation was introduced--the Tax Equity and Fiscal Responsibility Act--which included hospice under the Medicare benefit as detailed in Chapter 3's discussion of funding sources.

The Washington Business Group on Health (WBGH) was given the opportunity to comment on HHS regarding industry's potential role in the development of the hospice concept. Apparently, before business is willing and able to support hospice care, they must be provided with a sound data base. This would include the development of objective cost comparisons among existing hospice installations with studies showing the possible impact of authorized Medicare/Medicaid reimbursement for hospice services (Ross, 1978). The constructive participation of management and labor could vitally facilitate the development of criteria and guidelines for high quality flexible hospice care. At the same time, careful consideration must be taken to avoid many of the developmental and administrative errors that have occurred within both the Health Maintenance Organization (HMO) movement and Medicare and Medicaid Programs such as lack of physician support, organization deficiencies, poor management techniques, complex regulations, and limited funding.

Hospice, therefore, with some unique characteristics, is a timely health care reform which has the potential to bring about the necessary changes in the delivery of health care which the American public has desired for so long.

REFERENCES

Aries, Philippe. (1974). *Western Attitudes Toward Death.* Baltimore: Johns Hopkins University Press.

Brooks, Charles H., and Kathleen Smyth-Staruch. (1983). *Cost Savings of Hospice Home Care To Third-Party Insurers.* Cleveland, OH: Hospice Council for Northern Ohio, Blue Cross of Northeast Ohio, and Case Western Reserve University.

Califano, Joseph. (1978). Address to the National Hospice Organization's First Annual Banquet, Washington, DC, October 5th.

Cohen, Kenneth P. (1979). *Hospice Prescription for Terminal Care.* Rockville, MD: Aspen Systems Corporation.

Congressional Record. (1978). Intent description regarding terminal illness by Senators Edward M. Kennedy, Robert Dole, and Abraham Ribicoff. May 18th.

Cunningham, Robert Jr. (1979). When Enough is Enough. *Hospitals* 53(13): 63-65.

Dunphy, J. Engelbert. (1979). Rising Above Suffering and Death. *Bulletin of the American College of Surgeons* 64(4):10-11.

Glaser, Barney G., and Anselm L. Strauss. (1965). *Awareness of Dying.* Chicago: Aldine.

Goldenberg, Ira S. (1979). Hospice: To Humanize Dying. *Bulletin of the American College of Surgeons* 64(4):6-9.

Guthrie, Dorothea. (1979). Dr. Kubler-Ross: A Positive Acceptance of Death. *Bulletin of the American College of Surgeons* 64(4):12-13.

Halper, Thomas. (1979). On Death, Dying and Terminality: Today, Yesterday and Tomorrow. *Journal of Health Politics, Policy and Law* 4(1):11-29.

Hamilton, Michael, and Helen Reid. (1980). *A Hospice Handbook--A New Way To Care For The Dying.* Grand Rapids, MI: William B. Eerdmans Publishing Company.

Hendin, David. (1973). *Death as A Fact of Life.* New York: W. W. Norton and Co.

Kastenbaum, Robert J. (1977). *Death, Society, and Human Experience.* St. Louis: C. V. Mosby.

Kastenbaum, R., and R. Aisenberg. (1972). *The Psychology of Death.* New York: Springer.

Kubler-Ross, Elisabeth. (1969). *On Death and Dying.* New York: Macmillan.

_____. (1974). *Questions and Answers on Death and Dying.* New York: Macmillan.

_____. (1975). *Death: The Final Stage of Growth.* Englewood Cliffs, NJ: Prentice-Hall.

Mount, Balfour M. (1974). Death--A Fact of Life? *Crux* 11(3):6.

Munley, Anne. (1983). *The Hospice Alternative.* New York: Basic Books.

Munley, Anne, Cynthia S. Powers, and John B. Williamson. (1982). Humanizing Nursing Home Environments: The Relevance of Hospice Principles. *International Journal on Aging and Human Development* 15(4): 263-283.

Noyes, Russell Jr., and John Clancy. (1977). The Dying Role: Its Relevance To Improved Patient Care. *Psychiatry* 40:41-47.

Ross, Diane M. (1978). Medicine and Medicaid Hospice Projects. *Journal of American Insurance* 54(2):209.

Rossman, Parker. (1979). *Hospice.* New York: Fawcett Columbine.

Schoenberg, B., and A. C. Carr. (1972). *Psychosocial Aspects of Terminal Care.* New York: Columbia University Press.

Spiegel, Allen D. (1983). *Home Healthcare.* Owings Mills, MD: National Health Publishing.

Stoddard, Sandal. (1978). *The Hospice Movement.* Briarcliff Manor, NY: Stein and Day.

U.S. General Accounting Office. (1979). *Hospice Care--A Growing Concept in the United States.* HRD 79-50, March 6.

Wehr, Frederick T. (1980). *Toward a Gentler Dying Hospice Care In A General Hospital.* Baltimore: A. S. Abell Foundation.

Williamson, John B., Linda Evans, and Anne Munley. (1980). *Aging and Society.* New York: Holt, Rinehart and Winston.

Chapter 2

Hospice Implementation: Areas to Consider

In order to use the term hospice legitimately, a program must have certain essential characteristics. Hospice is more than a program of medical health care for the terminally ill; it is a model with specific, recognizable elements. Hospice care is characterized by its diversity; however, the modern hospice has certain distinctive features. Assumptions about resource "requirements" vary from program to program and are highly dependent on the philosophy, background, and skills of local hospice organizers. Specific standards of care distinguish hospice care from institutional and traditional home care and reflect the basis of hospice philosophy.

In this chapter we focus on fourteen points that should be considered; all relate in some way to critical components of a quality hospice program. Hospice leaders must have an in-depth understanding of each of these areas before planning and implementing a hospice program.

ADMINISTRATION AND COORDINATION OF SERVICES

Hospice must be an autonomous and centrally administered program which provides a continuum of care to the patient and family. Continuity of care reduces the patient's and the family's sense of alienation and fragmentation. Optimal utilization of services and resources is thus an important goal in the administration and coordination of patient care. A governing body (or designated persons) assumes full legal authority and responsibility for the operation of a hospice program. The governing body has written by-laws and oversees the administration, services, and fiscal management. A hospice program must have written and readily available evidence of its organization, services, and channels of authority for responsibility of the care provided to patients and their families.

Hospice programs seek to coordinate their services with professional and nonprofessional services in the community to avoid duplication of services and utilize existing resources as needed in the development of care plans. Appropriate referrals must be made for needed services beyond hospice care. Coordination requires both communication and leadership and must be evidenced in the organizational structure of each hospice model. Hospice programs must have defined affiliations, linkages, or arrangements for service with one or more facilities, service agencies, or programs along the continuum of care between acute inpatient, skilled and intermediate inpatient care, outpatient services, and home care services.

Professional management is the responsibility of hospice which includes the development and maintenance of central medical records and plans of care for hospice patients. Continuity of care is the presiding tenet and the patient/family benefit from one administrative representative for both home care and inpatient care.

Coordination and supervision by hospice staff for continuity among levels of care must be clearly written into hospice program policies. All professionals and supportive personnel involved in an individual's care become members of the hospice care team and follow the patient and family at whatever level of care is required. All team members must follow the hospice protocol and fully understand the plan of care. Management of the terminal illness is accomplished when the patient is in the appropriate setting based on need. With the ability of a hospice program to provide care in a variety of settings, the patient can enter the program and, if medically necessary, shift back and forth between settings without loss of continuity. Management of the care of hospice patients must always be retained by hospice caregivers who are trained and paid by hospice. Furthermore, any professional staff caring for the hospice patient in a hospital or skilled-nursing facility must be adequately trained by hospice educators. Coordination requires therapeutic communication among hospice staff and, in the case of a hospice patient in a hospital, the hospital staff become extended team members.

Supportive services, such as a required private duty nurse in the home to supplement the hospice care team, must also be trained by hospice educators. The traditional private duty nurse then becomes a member of the hospice care team assigned to a patient for a four- to eight-hour period of time. A quality educational program for interested health care professionals who agree to provide private duty type services to hospice patients is imperative. The ongoing inclusion of those individuals in the interdisciplinary group sessions secures a unified approach to the individual plan of care.

Flexibility and continuity are built into the hospice system of care. Flexibility in provision of hospice patient care is crucial due to the frequent changes in the patient's condition and the family's response to the progress of the disease. The key to successful coordination of inpatient-outpatient care is flexibility. The plan of care for each patient and family tries to provide continuity not only in regard to the plan of care, but also to the setting in which the care is provided, the time during which care is available, and the personnel who have contact with the patient and family. With such efforts to provide quality of life through continuity in these areas (services and personnel) it is hoped that the patient and family will not experience stress due to frequent changes of setting, personnel, or fragmentation of services.

And, most importantly, hospice care is available twenty-four hours a day, seven days a week. Since the needs of hospice patients and their families occur at any time, staff must always be available. Hospice care is intended to be flexible to meet the changing needs of the patient and family. Therefore, a hospice program of care makes its services available to every patient and family on the program whenever those services are needed. Emphasis is placed on the medical and nursing services being available around the clock in the home setting as well as the inpatient setting.

Overlapping of organizational and patient/family care goals can be accomplished through sound business management, excellent patient care, and a dedicated staff. Dynamic leadership, good staffing, budget flexibility, open communication channels, an active chief executive officer and board interest, democratic involvement in the management decision-making process, and freedom to grow all assure that the hospice program is a viable quality service to the community it serves.

PATIENT POPULATION

Age

Hospices serve patients ranging from the very young to the very old. Observed ranges are from age six to eighty-five. However, the average age is around sixty. Our research showed 67 percent of the aggregated patients over sixty-five, 16 percent in the fifty-five to sixty-four age group, 14 percent in the forty to fifty-four age group, and 3 percent in the twenty-one to thirty-nine age group. This confirms a pattern of older patients utilizing hospice services.

Age can assist in defining the types of services needed since each group requires a different focus on services and staff; for example, staff expertise in care of the geriatric patient is different from care of the child. The decision that a child has reached a terminal state is made more reluctantly. There is a tendency to "treat till the last" in the hope that something will work; consequently the time during which only symptomatic care is given may be relatively short. This may be why there are currently very few children in hospice programs. See Chapter 11 for further discussion of children and hospice.

Parents and siblings of ill and dying children suffer emotional stress that can affect many areas of their lives. Hospices must be sensitive to the feelings of the healthy siblings of a terminally ill child. The hospice concept of care can benefit these families. More than 100,000 children in the United States die annually. Children's Hospice International in Alexandria, Virginia was founded to address the issues surrounding hospice care for children and their families and to encourage the development of programs meeting the needs of seriously ill children and their families. Children's Hospice International promotes hospice support through pediatric care facilities, encourages the inclusion of children in existing and developing hospices and home care programs, includes the hospice perspectives in all areas of pediatric care and education, and makes the public aware of the needs of the seriously ill children and their families (Dailey, 1984). With this advocacy group the future should bring increased hospice services to children.

Sex

The sex of the patient is pertinent to program planning for some of the same reasons as age, that is, staffing and needed services. In the sites we studied, 57 percent of the patients were female and 43 percent were male. These statistics do have some effect on who the primary care person is and the amount of support which may be needed; for example, a male (with a terminally ill wife) often needs to continue working and may not be able to provide as much care; therefore, he would need additional supportive services from hospice. Without national statistics for comparison, patterns cannot be noted relating to sex. In 33 percent of the patients under age 65 in our study, medical record notations made by social workers stated that additional support services were necessary so the primary care person could continue working full time--in 57 percent of the patients the primary care person was a male spouse. The same was also noted for those partially retired individuals who continue working part time.

Diagnosis

Most programs have focused primarily upon terminal illness from malignant disease, although many have provided care to other types of patients, such as those with progressive neurological diseases, including multiple sclerosis and amyotrophic lateral sclerosis (ALS).

The literature confirms that hospices primarily serve terminal cancer patients and their families in those cases in which it is relatively easy to tell when a patient becomes terminal. Hospices, according to the comptroller's report, have also served a few patients in the terminal stage of kidney failure and heart disease (U.S. General Accounting Office, 1979).

One hospice program accepted three ALS patients in the beginning of their program who had an average length of stay of eighteen months. Because of this, the eligibility of patients is evaluated more comprehensively now than at the beginning of the program. Their appropriateness for the hospice program is certainly a big question--since they do represent a long-term chronic illness whose prognosis is difficult to evaluate. In contrast, another hospice program has expanded the eligibility requirement for admission to include the chronically ill patient--those with incurable, life-threatening, or lingering terminal illness. The hospice philosophy of care can be readily applied to the chronically ill individual who clearly has needs not met by our traditional health care delivery system. Hospice seems very appropriate as a program to fulfill that gap in some communities.

Therefore, hospice programs do vary as to criteria for admission. A recent survey in Pennsylvania shows 90 percent of the operating hospice programs admitting an individual with any terminal illness whereas, 10 percent admitted those with only a cancer diagnosis.

PROBABILITY OF HOME DEATH

The results of an Ohio research project (Brooks and Smyth-Staruch, 1983) support the claim that hospice home care programs shift the place of death from the hospital to the homes of cancer patients. Thirty-eight percent of the hospice cancer patients in that study died at home, as opposed to just 8 percent of nonhospice patients. Moreover, only 43 percent of the hospice cancer patients in the study died in a hospital, compared to 70 percent of the nonhospice patients. One of every five persons died in a nursing home among both hospice and nonhospice patients.

Since the focus for hospice care in the United States is in the home, one would expect that a patient and family admitted to a hospice program of care would remain in the home setting and the patient would die there. With patient and family education by the hospice care team, along with special hospice care and attention, the patient's chance of remaining at home until death is greater than without the benefit of a hospice program of care.

Experiences have shown that the objective of hospice programs to keep the patient at home with loved ones is not always met. A survey completed by the Pennsylvania Hospice Network based on 1983 patient data in 69 operating hospice *programs* in Pennsylvania which care for approximately 1,445 patients on a daily basis revealed that 56 percent of the patient deaths occurred at home. The remaining 44 percent died in an institution indicating the patient's condition required an acute or skilled care setting. (Pennsylvania Hospice Network, 1984). Our experiences have indicated that traditional home care agencies are not able to provide the extended hours of care as well as the level of care provided. The statistics in one home care model of hospice care showed only 32 percent of their hospice patients dying at home. The remaining 68 percent were hospitalized at the time of death. In the freestanding hospice, however, 84 percent of the patients die in the hospice itself, a facility providing services at that point in the illness. Fifty percent of the patients in the hospital-based model die at home as in the community model where the percentage varies from 55 to 63.

A close working relationship among caregivers is critical in planning the patient's location of death. The education of the patient's physician as to the objectives of the hospice program and the integration of the physician as a member of the hospice care team has a positive impact on keeping the patient at home. Frequently referrals are made with the approach that the patient/family prefer to stay at home if possible. However, we must be alert to the fact that some patients/families referred to hospice may elect hospitalization during a period of crisis.

Home care most frequently meets the needs of the dying person who has family to care for him. Additionally, it provides opportunity for the family to anticipate the loss of a member and to interact in an intimate and satisfying way.

The proverbial house can be put in order, business can be finished, and peace can be made as necessary (Jivaff, 1979).

Hospice caregivers frequently become concerned when hospice patients are hospitalized because they feel helping people to return to or remain at home is an important part of the hospice mission. Hospice personnel must be trained to accept and care for people where they are, since it is through personal contacts of this nature that the hospice program provides an image in the community as being a group of caring, helpful, and sensitive individuals.

RURAL AND URBAN HOSPICE PROGRAMS

The basic elements of a hospice are the same, whether it is located in an urban or rural area (Frickey, 1984). However, certain characteristics of rural communities present special concerns in the establishment of hospices and the acceptance of hospice concepts. In order to plan and develop effective hospice programs in rural areas, it is necessary to understand rural culture and the characteristics of rural communities. Rural and urban areas differ in style, customs, economic situation, population density, geographic location, and topography. According to Jenkins and Cook, (1981), people in rural areas are more similar to people in nonrural areas than they are different. Certain values and traditions are maintained in rural environments that tend to differentiate these areas from more populous areas. Rural Americans place a high value on the land, a closeness to the earth, a belief in the work ethic, a strong tendency toward insularity, a belief in the principle of self-help, an emphasis on family loyalty, and a tolerance for idiosyncratic behavior in members of the community. These attitudes do facilitate development of strong helping networks since formal service systems tend to be fragmented and located far from the hospice patient population. Formal and informal or natural helping systems can be integrated through a rural hospice program.

Recruitment of qualified staff, geographic distances between patients, the increased travel time from the central hospice office to patient homes, the small patient caseload due to lack of population density, communication problems due to increased mileage, and administration and coordination become critical concerns at a much more intensive level when implementing a rural hospice.

Government regulations for hospice benefits under Medicare originally specified that a hospice must routinely provide all core services--nursing, medical social services, physician services, and counseling. The regulations do provide for the use of contract staff to perform core services when peak patient loads or other extraordinary circumstances cause the hospice staffing needs to exceed normal staffing levels. Rural hospices have limitations in the recruitment of health care professionals since many rural communities have small numbers of registered nurses, medical social workers, physicians, and counselors available. Rural advocates were able to convince federal lawmakers of the staffing problems and lead them to understand the realities of how small, rural hospices must function. In 1984 federal officials provided a waiver on staffing regulations for rural hospices certified for hospice benefits under Medicare. The regulations stated that rural hospices in business before January 1, 1983 could obtain a waiver if the rural hospice administration could demonstrate that they had completed a good faith effort to hire their own nurses as opposed to contracting with the State Health Department or other agency or facility. Often rural hospices find it necessary to contract with the Health Department in order to assure the availability of professional nurses.

Geographic distances within a rural hospice require increased travel time and increased response time for home visits and ambulance calls, when required in an emergency. This increases the cost of care in comparison to an urban hospice. Smaller numbers of patients due to decreased population density limits hospice program development and staffing needs. Communication and coordination among hospice caregivers is difficult since telephone conferences warrant toll calls. Therapeutic communication among caregivers on a daily basis becomes a problem when members of the interdisciplinary team may be located in another county. A small caseload may not justify full-time staff including administrators and supervisors. In an urban hospice, the caseload is large enough to demand full-time administrators and caregivers.

A community education program for health care professionals and lay members must be carefully planned. Hospice advocates must understand and respect the existing provincialism in rural areas. Training seminars, lectures, classes, and group presentations can be effective only with involvement of the community members in the initial planning and implementation. The close ties within a small town where neighbors, friends, and relatives are genuinely concerned about one another and wish to assist in the event of illness and stress present positive aspects for a hospice program. These relationships provide a base to build upon in planning a supportive hospice program for the terminally ill patient and family. In this respect, a volunteer program in a rural area often has its beginning with those individuals who are committed to caring for neighbors and friends.

The traditional older rural resident has established a lifestyle of self-sufficiency and self-reliance. Family members are usually cared for at home until a crisis develops that warrants hospitalization. The alternative, a flexible hospice home care program, can improve the quality of life for the entire community. Volunteer services coordinated by an existing service or facility are frequently the mainstay of rural hospices. The interdisciplinary team members may not be as diverse as in urban hospices but, nevertheless, they are fully able to provide a range of hospice services. Five hundred out of 1,500 hospice programs are in rural areas. Although state hospice organizations are addressing concerns and issues in rural hospices, research needs to be undertaken to identify problems specific to these communities.

HOSPICE FUNDING AND INSURANCE COVERAGE

An important aspect of hospice care is that services are provided based on need rather than the patient's or family's ability to pay. Before third-party reimbursement was instituted in November 1983, hospice programs were reimbursed in the manner of traditional programs. If the existing reimbursement structure did not cover hospice care, services were paid for by the patient and family themselves or through various contributions. Limited federal and state grants for research demonstrations and pilot projects assisted in supporting fledgling hospice organizations.

Reimbursement for hospice-type home care is more complex because the length of the visit is two to three times longer than a traditional home care visit. Also, bereavement and spiritual services are not reimbursable separately though they are a crucial part of hospice care.

The seeking of funding sources is discussed fully in Chapter 3. If, through a regular, consistent source of income, programs were able to achieve a greater measure of financial stability, hospice administrators could create a regular staff of accountable personnel and expand hospice services in the community.

Blue Cross/Blue Shield have shown an interest in the incorporation of hospice care into the total health care delivery system. Negotiations have led to the establishment of various "pilot" hospice programs but since each Blue Cross/Blue Shield plan is autonomous, hospices have had to contact them individually to discuss reimbursement.

The Medicare Hospice Benefit currently provides third-party reimbursement for certified hospices. Under the Tax Equity and Fiscal Responsibility Act (TEFRA) of 1982, provisions for hospice care were authorized with a "sunset" provision so the hospice benefit will be available only from November 1, 1983 through September 30, 1986. Congress expanded the Medicare (Part A) hospital insurance program to include hospice care as a new benefit for three years which began November 1, 1983. This means that people who have a terminal illness can now receive a full scope of medical and support services for their terminal condition while continuing to live in their own homes or other settings outside of a hospital. The special rules that apply to Medicare coverage of, and payment for, hospice care are summarized as follows:

1. Under Medicare, hospice is primarily a comprehensive home care program which provides all the reasonable and necessary medical and support services for the management of a terminal illness, including pain control. Covered services include physician services, nursing care, medical appliances and supplies (including outpatient drugs for symptom management and pain relief), home health aide and homemaker services, therapies, medical social services, and counseling. In addition to the broad range of outpatient services, short-term inpatient care is also covered. When a patient receives these services from a Medicare-certified hospice, Medicare hospital insurance pays almost the entire

cost. There are no deductibles or copayments, except for limited cost-sharing for outpatient drugs and inpatient respite care.

2. to be eligible for hospice care, four conditions must be met:

- the patient is eligible for Medicare (Part A) hospital insurance;

- the patient's doctor and the hospice medical director certify that the patient has a terminal illness;

- the patient signs a statement choosing hospice care instead of standard Medicare benefits for the terminal illness;

- the patient receives care from a Medicare-certified hospice program.

3. Hospice services can be provided by a public agency or private organization that is primarily engaged in furnishing care to terminally ill people and their families. To receive Medicare payment, the agency or organization must be certified by Medicare to provide hospice services--even if it is already approved by Medicare to provide other kinds of health services. The patient's doctor at the particular organization or agency selected for hospice care can tell the patient whether its program is approved by Medicare. Information about Medicare-certified hospice programs in local areas is also available from Social Security offices.

4. Special benefit periods apply to hospice care. A patient can receive hospice care for two periods of ninety days each and one thirty-day period--a lifetime maximum of 210 days. If hospice care is chosen for the terminal condition but later the patient decides not to use it, he or she can cancel at any time and resume standard hospital and medical insurance benefits under Medicare Part A and Part B. If cancellation is made before the end of a hospice period, any days left in that period are forfeited, but the patient is still eligible for any remaining hospice periods. For example: if a patient cancels at the end of sixty days in the first ninety-day period, he or she loses the remaining thirty days. However, the patient is still eligible at a future time for the second ninety-day period and one thirty-day period. A patient can change from one hospice program to another once during each period without canceling the hospice care.

If a patient continues to need services after the hospice benefit periods are exhausted, the hospice must continue providing care unless the patient no longer wants hospice services.

5. Medicare pays the hospice directly for the full cost of all of the reasonable and necessary covered services it provides for a terminal illness and related health problems. There are no deductibles or copayments, except for two items:

- Drugs or biologicals for pain relief and symptom management: The hospice can charge 5 percent of the reasonable cost, up to a maximum of five dollars, for each outpatient prescription for pain relief and symptom management.

● Inpatient respite care: During a hospice period a patient may need short-term inpatient care to enable the person who regularly assists to get some temporary relief. This is called respite care for which the hospice can charge 5 percent of the cost of the inpatient stay, up to a total of $356 (1984 amount). The patient may not be charged more than this amount during a period that begins when a hospice plan is first chosen and ends fourteen days after such care is canceled. (Respite care is limited each time to stays of no more than five days in a row).

6. Since Medicare hospital insurance (Part A) covers the full cost of all medical and support services for a terminal condition, the patient gives up the right to payment for standard Medicare benefits for the terminal illness when hospice care is chosen. However, there are two exceptions:

● If a patient's attending physician is not working for the hospice, Medicare medical insurance (Part B) continues to pay for his or her services in the same way it usually pays for other doctor's services. Medicare pays for 80 percent of the approved amount for covered services after the annual Part B deductible is met.

● Medicare continues to cover treatment for conditions other than the terminal illness, under standard Medicare benefits.

All other services must be provided by or through the hospice.

7. When care from a hospice is chosen, Medicare cannot pay for:

● Treatment for the terminal illness which is not for symptom management and pain control;

● Care provided by any other hospice (unless the patient's hospice arranged it).

● Care from another provider which is the same as, or duplicates, care the hospice is required to provide. (Department of Health and Human Services, 1984).

8. As of November 1, 1983 payment amounts were established to reimburse specific categories of covered hospice care based on national rates with an aggregate cap limitation of $6,500 per patient.

● Routine home care day ($46.25)

● Continuous home care day ($358.67)

● Inpatient respite care day ($55.33)

● General inpatient care day ($271.00)

On November 9, 1984, President Reagan signed a law increasing the reimbursement rate for routine home care under Medicare from $46.25 to $53.17 effective October 1, 1984.

The final regulations have placed a limitation on inpatient care by specifying that a hospice must assure that it does not exceed 20 percent of the aggregate number of days of hospice care provided to Medicare beneficiaries during any twelve-month period (Department of Health and Human Services, 1983). A further discussion of this benefit is detailed in Chapter 3 where the author highlights the potential for viability. An existing reimbursement system must be established to keep the program viable.

In order for services to be available to everyone, hospice administrators must continue to advocate for increased funding services and seek to change regulations which stifle the provision of hospice services. The determination of costs and the financial viability of any hospice care program should begin with a look at standards of care. Acceptable standards for hospice care are of utmost concern to the public and to those committed to implementing the hospice concept without compromising its philosophy. Since standards of care require delineation of resources necessary for hospice care, recognition and acceptance of minimum standards is a basic financial consideration. However, there is no present consensus on either minimal or optimal acceptable standards. Hospitals have ready means to meet high standards in a cost-effective and efficient manner through program management and through Joint Commission for Accreditation of Hospitals (JCAH). JCAH is now aggressively promoting its hospice accreditation program. This is discussed further in Chapter 4. Fluctuating hospice census and varying intensity of services are managed with maximum productivity through program-oriented plans and goals superimposed over existing departmental structures to allow effective staffing.

The funds received from grants, endowments, or other special trust sources such as memorials are useful in underwriting start-up expenses, but generally cannot be relied upon for continued operational support on a large scale. As with other forms of health care, third-party reimbursement comprises the major source of operating funds. Since this reimbursement system categorizes health care services according to levels, hospice care is reimbursed according to services approved under acute (hospital), skilled/intermediate (nursing home) or home care levels. Third-party reimbursement is generally not sufficient to cover the labor intensive expense of hospice patients. However, major components of hospice care do fall within reimbursement guidelines and provide a foundation for the survival of a program. Third-party reimbursement does not cover such program components as pastoral care, bereavement follow-up, respite care, and many professional consultative services. However, Title XX* funds are beginning to cover counseling and homemaker services to those eligible under the age of sixty. Hospice programs have found it necessary to carry out their

---

* Later known as Adult Block Grants

bereavement program through use of volunteers for economic reasons. Volunteers who are going to serve as lay therapists or group facilitators require additional training in the areas of the hospice concept, bereavement theory, and needs of widowed persons. Sixty-five percent of hospice patients are covered for skilled services under Medicare. This is clearly expected based on the higher percentage of over age sixty-five patients. The resources of self-paying patients are often sorely taxed by the costs of prolonged illness and/or the aggressive curative treatment which usually precedes hospice care. The savings potential of hospice care is primarily a matter of providing an alternative to expensive acute care technology as well as decreasing the length of stay which is currently being demonstrated in the hospital-based inpatient unit. Savings are more significant if one assumes that the alternative for many terminally ill cancer patients is an intensive battery of expensive curative measures more costly than those used by the average patient. While it is encouraging to find evidence of cost efficiency, it is of little value unless the program meets its objectives and standards.

HOSPICE EDUCATION: TRAINING PROGRAMS

Hospice staff and volunteers must participate in an organized educational program which provides orientation and ongoing training for hospice care. Initially each potential staff person should be required to attend the volunteer training program. Upon successful completion of this program, the individual can then be considered for employment.

Continuing education is also important. There is a continual need to improve the techniques of palliative care and to disseminate such information. Because there is a practical limit to the amount of individual attention that can be offered in the initial orientation, hospice programs need to set up a basic instructional course that includes some group instruction supplemented by one-to-one instruction in the unit or in the home care situation. The educational program extends beyond the hospice care team into the community.

Funding resources for education are also necessary in program development. Staff must be provided access to in-service programs while on paid time whenever possible. Chapter 3 discusses further the development of hospice education programs.

Hospice educational philosophy introduces the potential team member to the hospice program of care and promotes good interpersonal relations and effective communication within the hospice community.

The principles of this philosophy include the following:

- Progress is made through the acquisition of new knowledge.

- Training is an ongoing process and hospice is responsible for the continued education of its staff.

- The program depends on the ability of all staff members to do their job efficiently, which can only be accomplished with an effective educational program.

- An effective educational program which stimulates the staff interest in self-improvement results in all-around improvement of care.

- The establishment of any effective program must consider the personal, psychological, and social needs of the trainees as well as their professional, scientific, or technical needs.

- Opportunity for professional and personal development, made possible through an effective educational program, will result in increased job satisfaction, motivation, and high staff morale.

- The educational program coordinates both staff and program needs enhancing value and services to patients and their families.

- The educational program is based on adequate and realistic determination of learning needs as well as the setting of realistic objectives to meet these needs, and results in behavioral changes to meet those objectives.

Hospice's education program is formalized, centralized, coordinated, and directed toward the needs of the total organization with effective use of resources, including people, facilities, and funds. There is a continuous conscious effort to assist the hospice care team to meet needs for self-esteem, growth, and satisfaction. Cooperation, collaboration, and sharing among members of the hospice care team in program assessment, planning, implementation, and evaluation is essential for assurance of quality care for the patient and his or her family.

The orientation and development of skills through ongoing in-service education are components of the overall educational program. This includes:

- Documentation of courses, classes, seminars, and so on with a brief description of content, objectives, methods of learning, and criteria for evaluation.

- Content directed at the level of the learner consistent with the scope of assignment.

- Behavioral objectives.

- Supervised clinical practice integrated with theory.

The orientation program is focused on teaching hospice philosophy, program components, policies, and procedures. The educational program is a competency-based program utilizing an assessment tool to determine skills and abilities. The orientation program is then individualized to assist hospice care team members gain specialized skills and abilities. The concept of competency-based orientation is implemented through use of an appropriate preceptor, for example, nursing or medical social work. A skill inventory checklist determines the amount of skills required.

The hospice RN and MSW clinical and educational supervisors carry out the orientation and ongoing educational program assigning each staff member to an individual preceptor (supervisor) to help in development of skills. Orientation activities must be documented on a specified form kept in the staff personnel folder.

Hospice promotes the continuing education of staff members and advisors. By operating within the annual budgetary guidelines, the administrator, board of directors, and staff select the education program(s) that they deem will be most beneficial to agency progress. The board of directors will also provide time off for staff members so that they may be able to attend the seminar(s). Attendance at all seminars and meetings is documented in personnel files.

In addition, monthly educational programs are conducted. Staff are requested to attend on a paid-time basis. These include the following as documented in the form of minutes and on specific forms in the in-service manual on a monthly basis:

- monthly program on selected topics;

- staff support meetings coordinated and directed by coordinator of bereavement services;

- clinical conference with medical director;

- clinical oncology meetings at the local hospital with clinical team members from hospice and the local hospital;

- other coordinated staff conferences based on need.

- Hospice's written coordinated plan for staff education must include sources of funding and time off for attendance.

Hospice staff must be encouraged to attend professional meetings such as the annual National Hospice Organization meeting and to participate in continuing education programs and activities which will expand their knowledge and skills. At the discretion of the executive committee of the board of directors, time off should be given to attend selected meetings, and all reasonable expenses for attendance at professional meetings should be reimbursed. In addition, a hospice course offered in local educational institutions is a very effective mechanism for reaching a wider population.

Hospice courses also need to be included in the curriculum of colleges on both an undergraduate and graduate level, primarily specialty areas such as gerontology, health services administration, nursing, and social work.

EVALUATION OF HOSPICE SERVICES

Evaluation of hospice services is an ongoing activity in a hospice care program. In order for a hospice program to reach its full potential, careful evaluation should be done for the overall program, the individual hospice patients, and for individual hospice staff. The precise method of evaluation is an individual matter depending upon the particular program. Hospice programs should be evaluated for the reasons listed below:

1. To demonstrate to other groups that the hospice program is an effective health care program

2. To justify past or projected expenditures

3. To determine costs

4. To gain support for expansion of facilities

5. To determine future objectives

6. To determine program efficiency

7. To assure quality of care

8. To assist in ongoing development and assessment of adequate staffing patterns and staff qualifications

9. To prepare for certification. Evaluation for hospice staff can be a time for honest feedback and creative sharing. It is a time for setting goals and voicing expectations for the immediate future. Evaluation is an essential component of health care today; it forces programs to assess their organization, staff, services, and finances.

The delivery of hospice care requires periodic appraisals by board and staff representatives and professional people outside the hospice program serving on hospice advisory committees and working in conjunction with consumers. The overall program evaluation approach includes a review of the hospice programs and services, a review of administrative and fiscal management, review of policies, analysis of statistics, and review of all records.

Activities performed by hospice caregivers and committees associated with the agency are guidelines to help determine the appropriateness, quantity, and quality of service. The outcome of these activities identifies areas within the total program that show growth and those that need improvement and/or change. Program evaluation helps all hospice caregivers recognize that the outcomes of their activities are significant to and interrelated with the achievement of the overall program goals. Participation in program evaluation assists members of the hospice team to assume responsibility for evaluation of their own professional activities as part of the total program evaluation. Self-evaluation is useful, therefore, in:

- identifying program strengths and weaknesses
- determining direction to take in improving, expanding, and developing hospice care
- indicating areas where consultation may be needed
- orienting hospice staff to hospice organization and administration, including fiscal management, as well as patient care
- interpreting services and community needs to advisory committees and others in the community
- reviewing the efficiency and effectiveness of the total hospice program
- observing patient outcomes

Program evaluation will be further discussed in Chapter 4 in terms of quality assurance in hospice implementation and practice. The development of a tool or guide to assist in the evaluation of the total program is significant. This mechanism allows hospice programs to prepare for licensure, certification, or accreditation in meeting the conditions of participation. The emphasis must focus on quality and outcome as well as structure and process.

PALLIATIVE VERSUS CURATIVE CARE

In the hospice context, palliative treatment is the relief of pain and other troubling symptoms by appropriate coordination of all elements of care needed to achieve relief from distress. The goal of hospice care is to provide symptom control through appropriate palliative therapies. Symptom control includes assessing and responding to the physical, emotional, social, and spiritual needs of the patient/family.

The conventional approach to care includes the continuing of therapies and life support systems, whereas, the focus of hospice care is symptomatic treatment only, such as radiation therapy for reduction in tumor size, nerve blocks for relief of pain, or administration of oxygen to ease breathing but not to prolong life. Palliative care is an appropriate form of care when cure is no longer possible. The goal of palliative care is the prevention of distress from chronic signs and symptoms such as pain. Pain medication should be ordered on a regular basis around the clock. When signs and symptoms are continuous, palliative therapies should be administered routinely to prevent the reemergence of symptoms that interfere with comfortable living. The goal of pain control therapy is not to induce an artificial state of euphoria, but to produce a state of physical and mental relief so that the patient can live and relate to others as normally as possible. Such care should neither hasten nor postpone death. Continual and careful monitoring is required to maintain such pain control, an important part of hospice care.

In conventional practice, pain is treated with limited medication on an as-necessary basis. Physicians and nurses fear psychological dependence and addiction; their goal is treatment, not prevention of pain. Studies show that addiction is not a factor in chronic pain, if pain is continually prevented and the dose is just enough to eliminate it. Careful and continual titration of the amount of narcotic to individual need is monitored and prescribed for administration at regular intervals around the clock to eliminate pain and the fear of recurrence of pain, while maintaining normal effect. Ease of administration is emphasized for patient mobility and independence. Within hospice the emphasis is on relief of side effects of narcotics, especially constipation and nausea.

Palliative care is the appropriate approach for hospice patients. This is based on the rationale that good palliative care for the patient who has no hope for cure should be a part of the continuum of the patient's medical care. Palliation can also be viewed as a hopeful, realistic goal, demonstrating that more can be done to comfort the patient. A medical record audit showed treatments and medication orders for symptom control as follows:

- Oxygen for difficult breathing

- Compazine for nausea

- Ferrasequela for weakness

- Tigan suppositories to relieve nausea

- Physical therapy for advice on maintaining balance

- Medication for swollen legs and feet, nutritional supplements for dehydration, medication for depression

- T.E.N.* in constant use for pain control

- Vitamin C for anemia, weakness, loss of appetite, and poor color

- Medication to control infection

- Stress tab. for stress relief

- Codeine for cough

- Ducolax, colace, glycerine suppositories, and other medications for constipation

- Valium for anxiety

---

* T.E.N.--transcutaneous electrical nerve stimulation--it is a device used directly on area of pain. It is supervised by a physical therapist team member.

- Dalmane for sleeplessness
- Elavil for depression
- Aspirin for bone pain inflammation
- Prednisolone for soft tissue swelling
- Xylocaine viscous for throat pain
- Mycostatin swish for sore mouth
- Lemon and glycerine swabs for sore mouth
- Varied approaches to decubiti care; for example, Betadine peroxide irrigation, Maalox, preventive measures such as turning to decrease pressure and keeping area clean and dry

Antitumor therapy for palliative purposes is available for hospice patients. Antitumor therapy in the form of surgery, radiation, chemotherapy, and endocrine manipulation is employed only insofar as it contributes to palliation. The purpose of such palliation is to relieve distressing symptoms quickly and thus improve the quality of the remaining life.

Easy availability of X-ray and other diagnostic mechanisms necessary for determining treatment needed for the patient's comfort is indicated for hospice patients. Advanced malignancy commonly affects many organs in the body and disturbs the biochemical balance. Terminal care must involve careful attention to the multitude of symptoms which a patient may therefore develop in his or her last weeks or months of life. As in general medicine, it is important to diagnose the cause of each symptom and to base treatment on it. A medical record audit by this author evidenced how one patient had a colostomy performed for relief of obstructive symptoms, another patient had an intramedullary nail inserted to prevent further pathological fractures, and another patient had hemorrhoids removed to relieve symptoms.

Pain and symptom control are extremely important in the care of hospice patients underscoring the philosophy that if pain and symptoms are not under reasonable control, other comfort and caring measures are usually fruitless and may even be counterproductive.

COMBATING DEHUMANIZATION

Hospice is viewed as a humanizing mode of health care which has the capacity to enhance quality of life. Hospice emphasizes patient individuality and responsiveness to the total needs of the dying person and his or her family. Hospice has the potential to provide a social context for humane, personalized death in which maximum effort can be made to control pain in all its forms: physical, psychological, social, and spiritual (Munley, Powers, and Williamson, 1982).

Terminal patients are frequently isolated--separated from patients expected to live and from their families, sometimes even deserted by their physicians. In the inpatient setting nurses take longer to answer these patients' bells. Within the hospice program, presence and companionship are considered essential; communication and support are emphasized. Hospice inpatient care includes more than normal nursing hours per patient per day with volunteer assistance. Families participate actively in the care of their loved one. Families stay overnight during crisis periods in the hospice setting. Hospice offers unlimited visiting hours; and children are permitted to visit as well.

Treatment with high technology is a central feature of conventional health care delivery: physical systems are maintained with intravenous fluids, forced feedings, and nasogastric tubes; laboratory examinations, and X-rays are routinely performed. In most instances, all such measures are discontinued in hospice since they are unnecessary and do not contribute to the comfort of the patient. Primary concerns for hospice patients are comfort, mobility, and active participation in their lives. Traditionally, little attention was directed to treatment of the patient's diminishing resources and self-confidence as disease and disfigurement progress. In hospice care the greatest possible feeling of well-being and self-worth is promoted. Physical, occupational, speech, music, drama, art, and recreational therapies are employed.

Hospice places emphasis on the patient as a person and family member. Patients are encouraged to express individuality, wear their own clothes, eat foods they like, and maintain their own idiosyncrasies. Hospice patients are allowed to die as they lived, not according to a predetermined mold.

The hospice environment considers the inherent worth and individuality of each person. Hospice staff recognizes each patient's need for privacy and personal autonomy; the establishment of mutual respect is fundamental to hospice principles.

The hospice model is characterized by its belief in the right of the individual patient to make prime decisions with respect to his or her care.

PATIENT AND FAMILY AS A UNIT OF CARE

The hospice patient and family are treated together as a unit of care. Families undergo significant stress during the terminal illness of one of their members. If this stress is not acknowledged and therapeutically addressed, significant physical, emotional, social, and spiritual disorders can result. Staff from hospice programs should be available to spend time, provide information, share insights and reactions, and assist in referrals as necessary for families in need. Families have a right to know the specific details of their situation and that of the dying member, so that they may prepare for death and take full advantage of present opportunities. Hospice staff identify the patient's family as persons who are legally related and also those persons regarded as significant by the patient.

The psychological and social problems that confront both the patient and the patient's family are often more distressing than the disease itself. Depression and anxiety are problems of relatives as well as patients. Family members often deny their own needs while caring for the terminally ill loved one. The hospice team is attentive to family members' feelings of neglect and resentment, as well as such feelings in the patient.

Frequently, the family can provide valuable information to the professionals on details of care. They may provide explanations of certain expressions unique to the patient. They may provide information on the frequency of medication or which positions the patient finds more comfortable. The hospice caregivers encourage family participation in patient care and provide support for them. Active participation by family members is part of the process of separation. Family members who are actively involved in the process of care while the patient is alive adjust to life without the patient after death more readily than those not involved (Munley, 1983).

Most importantly, the hospice care team acknowledges and respects the fact that each patient/family has its own beliefs and/or value system.

Family is referred to in its very broadest sense and includes the spouse, children, parents, uncles, aunts, cousins, neighbors, and friends. Often, a patient's closest interpersonal relationships are with individuals who are not related by blood or marriage and who become the primary care person. As family understanding and acceptance grows, the family is used as a part of the therapeutic team.

HOSPICE INTERDISCIPLINARY TEAM

The hospice care concept employs the interdisciplinary (IDG) team as opposed to the multidisciplinary team. The interdisciplinary approach requires that the team members from different disciplines integrate and coordinate their caregiving efforts rather than function independently in caring for the patient. Interdisciplinary care is a carefully planned effort involving professionals, family, close friends, and volunteers. This type of care is based on a belief that no one person can handle all the needs of the dying patient; hospice seeks to meet those needs as completely and humanely as possible.

The core team should consist of the patient's family, the attending physician, and hospice personnel, such as physician, oncologist, psychiatrist, nurse, social worker, therapies such as physical, speech, occupational, respiratory, patient care coordinator, volunteer coordinator, pharmacist, nutritionist, and clergy. Other special services should be available such as medical, paramedical, legal, financial, religious, e.g., enterostomal therapy, specialty medical evaluations, mental health counseling, bereavement counseling, art therapy, music therapy, pastoral counseling, and assistance by volunteers. No one individual or professional can meet all the needs of terminally ill patients and families all the time. Every member of the hospice interdisciplinary patient care team recognizes the value of his or her own particular level of expertise, in either a professional or personal capacity, for meeting at least one aspect of a patient and family's needs with the awareness that each discipline relates with other disciplines in the delivery of the overall plan of care to the patient. This results in what is often referred to as "role blurring." The hospice program seeks to provide a community of care for patients and families dealing with the distress of terminal illness. The strength of the interdisciplinary team in this regard is that all members of the team have a common commitment to meet the patient's and family's needs, and this commitment supersedes the boundaries of their own disciplines. They not only contribute on the basis of their own expertise but they also give other team members insight into their own fields. For example, a nurse may become involved with developing and delivering social service aspects of care; the physician may perform nursing care; a volunteer may respond to spiritual questions, and so on. The team trains, encourages, and supports itself in the delivery of such a blending of professional and nonprofessional services.

Since symptoms come from a variety of sources--physical, psychological, social, spiritual, financial, and legal--physicians, nurses, social workers, physical therapists, nutritionist, clergy, lawyers, and volunteers are all important components of a hospice care program. Advanced malignancy brings with it a variety of problems. In addition, the patient and his family bring to the terminal illness all of the baggage of life, including preexisting personality, marital, and financial problems. In coping with all of these complexities, a team approach is important; it can draw upon professional expertise from a variety of fields in order to resolve difficulties. Furthermore, patients are highly individual in their ability to relate to other people; therefore, the availability of many team members provides the opportunity for support from a number of sources. According to Zimmerman (1981), it is this feature of hospice that serves as the enabling link between the kind of personal attention which the family physician could provide and the sophisticated techniques of modern health care. There are few circumstances left in which it is possible for physician and nurse to provide the breadth and depth of care which a well-organized hospice care team can offer.

In practice, the IDG team--composed of hospice employees and known as the hospice care team--provides and supervises the care and services offered by hospice. Altogether, the team consists of one or more medical directors, registered nurses, medical social workers, enterostomal therapists, pastoral care counselors, a dietary counselor, licensed practical nurses, home health aides, social work assistants, physical therapists, a speech therapist, an occupational therapist, a respiratory therapist, volunteers, a pharmacist, a psychiatrist, a bereavement counselor, and an art, music, and drama therapist.

The hospice care team members meet weekly to review and update the plan of care of each patient/family. In addition, daily communication is ongoing among the team members. The hospice care team assesses and reviews in detail the plan of care for each patient/family unit upon admission and again no later than seven days after admission to the hospice program. The clinical record and minutes of weekly meetings must document involvement of all team members.

The core services--doctor of medicine, registered nurse, social worker, pastoral counselor, and dietary counselor--are the interdisciplinary group with primary responsibility of provision and supervision of care. This supervision by the IDG establishes the plan of care prior to providing care and reviews the plan of care weekly, but no longer than every two weeks. The IDG also participates in the establishment of policies governing the day-to-day provision of hospice care and services.

Services provided by the interdisciplinary team are coordinated by a registered nurse and medical social worker to assure ongoing assessment of the patient's and family's needs and implementation of the interdisciplinary team care plan. The provision of care by each interdisciplinary team service is documented and is representative of current standards of practice for every interdisciplinary team service.

PASTORAL CARE

The spiritual needs and concerns of human beings are considered important in hospice care. Pastoral counseling is included as a component of the health care plan.

The importance of the clergy as a member of the hospice team is based on the conviction that personal, philosophical, moral, or religious belief systems are important to patients and families who face death. Hospice pastoral care is respectful of all patient and family belief systems, and will use all possible resources to meet individual needs. Thus, trained clergy must be available for patients and their families if they desire. For many, the acceptance of an impending death can be aided through religious and spiritual comfort. Such comfort may assist both the patient and his family to cope with feelings of anger and guilt, as well as provide a more meaningful context for life and death.

Members of the hospice pastoral care department function as an integral component of all caregiving. Careful planning and coordination of its service with local ministries and other disciplines within the hospice team is essential and accomplished through the interdisciplinary team process. The IDG pastoral care member respects the personal affiliations of a patient and his or her family, and develops working relations with community clergy of all faiths to foster their cooperation and collaboration in care.

The pastoral care team members provide support to assuage that spiritual pain that often enters the lives of persons facing a life-threatening illness together (Connecticut Hospice, Inc., 1984). The pastoral care department provides religious services which reflect an ecumenical approach. The memorial services which are held as a component of the bereavement support services also involve the pastoral care department. In addition, the role of the pastoral care department includes consultation, referral, and education.

The essence of spiritual caregiving is not doctrine or dogma but the capacity to enter into the world of the other and to respond with feeling. The hospice fosters such caregiving because it legitimates expressive role behavior, emphasizes respect for patient individuality, and creates a work climate in which staff members have time for personal relationships with patients (Munley, 1983).

Traditionally, spiritual support for the terminally ill is relegated to clergy and chaplains who are not always particularly skilled in this area. Each hospice team member, therefore, is responsive to spiritual matters. Openness and acceptance of the patients "where they are" rather than "where they should be" is the hospice approach, with participation of all team members, not clergy alone. Spiritual counseling or pastoral care, therefore, can be broadly defined as the efforts by all staff to help persons in their spiritual quest for wholeness and dignity. In this sense, all the activities of the hospice team can be included under the term "spiritual."

VOLUNTEER SERVICES

Volunteer services are an important component of the hospice program, and volunteers are made available and assigned as needed by a coordinator. The extent to which volunteers are available can affect the degree of service provided to each hospice patient, as well as the hospice's costs. If they are carefully selected, trained volunteers contribute invaluable warmth and skills in enhancing and supplementing many areas of patient comfort. Not only does the volunteer offer a perspective that is different from what a professional can achieve, but the presence of volunteers makes it possible to offer some services that could not otherwise be provided. Volunteers perform varied tasks in the home for patients and families. Volunteers can assist with meals, help to make beds, do light household chores, simply sit with a patient to provide companionship or time off for a primary caregiver, visit bereaved families, or help to run support groups for survivors. Volunteers can also provide transportation, run errands, assist in obtaining equipment for patients, do grocery shopping, read to patients and perform any other activities to assist in the patient's comfort. Volunteers help to alter clothes, some fix hair, some make wheelchair ramps, and some just sit and listen. The task is to explore carefully the needs of those who are being served and to respond to those needs in an imaginative way. Those who do not wish to be involved in patient care may render clerical services in the volunteer office.

In general, the hospice volunteer becomes more involved in direct patient care activities than the traditional hospital volunteer who delivers mail and flowers or acts as a hostess in the intensive care unit waiting room. Hospice volunteers are integrated and respected as members of the hospice caregiving team. Volunteers augment hospice work by providing their extra resources, maximizing the quality of care. Patients and families continue to tell us it is often the volunteer who makes the difference in quality.

Hospice care consists of a blending of volunteer and professional services in order to meet the ongoing needs of patients and families. Volunteers should be used as an integral part of the health care team. The volunteer program can offer a valuable supportive service when organized effectively. The lay or professional person who contributes time and talent to hospice without economic remuneration is a very special person who can be productive in a very efficient and effective caregiving manner with quality concerns.

Some staff members, especially nurses and social workers, first came to hospice programs as volunteers and went through the hospice's volunteer training course aiding mutual understanding. Nurses and social workers frequently offer their professional services voluntarily. Potential hospice staff go through the training program as volunteers and study with the volunteers, gaining respect for their services. The lay volunteers also come to learn and respect the professional's role.

Volunteers can come from the community-at-large and can be trained in usable skills. Most volunteers are students, housewives, senior citizens, and are usually unemployed. Such volunteers generally come in with some skills. Some of the services provided by hospice volunteers include the offer of respite to regular caregivers, errand-running such as to a drug store or supermarket, meal preparation, recreational services such as playing cards, going to a movie, companionship, delivery, homemaking, nutritional and other education, primary care person (PCP) relief, transportation, inpatient services, clerical work, committee and conference participation, and public speaking. The role of the volunteer has not been immune to questions about quality of care. Some hospice programs use the term "hospice assistant" rather than "volunteer" to suggest a function distinct and apart from that of the traditional hospital volunteer. The main role of the hospice assistant is to give the patient and family an opportunity to spend as much time with their loved ones as possible; to help reduce stress caused by tension and frustration; to provide the patient and family with a feeling of warmth and understanding at this transitional stage of their life, and during the period of bereavement. Through a volunteer support program, staffing expenses can be defrayed. This is especially true in the context of hospice care standards, where personal attention and time to spend with the patient and family must be readily available. However, in order for volunteer support to be meaningful from both a quality and financial standpoint, it must be incorporated into program planning and be consistently available.

The arrangement of volunteer relationships with patients tends to follow one of two patterns. In most home care situations, the entire hospice team-- which includes volunteers--is responsible for patients but one member coordinates the care and handles interteam communications; volunteers see the patients as needed. In the inpatient setting, the volunteers work in shifts, caring for patients for a set period of hours on a somewhat fixed schedule. Some patients can leave the inpatient setting and return home; to avoid disruption of the patient-volunteer relationship, the volunteer continues to communicate with, and often visit, the patient at home. In both models, continuity of the relationship between the patient and the volunteer is paramount. This continuity is as important for the patient's family as for the patient, and does not end with the patient's death.

It is essential to employ a paid volunteer director to maintain a stable and well-organized volunteer staff. This is discussed further in Chapter 3 in the section on program development.

Volunteers do not replace paid positions; they provide additional services which enhance the care of families and augment the work of paid staff in all departments. Quality service is more important than large rosters of volunteers or quantity of hours.

Volunteers must understand the total hospice program before beginning service. Each volunteer is placed in a job that best utilizes his or her skills and individuality. This encourages commitment, job satisfaction, and a sense of effective integration into the hospice community. Volunteer service is consistent with hospice goals and with standards set for paid personnel. Hospice volunteers today are the strength of hospice service delivery systems. They enrich the patients' extended family life and build bridges to the community.

BEREAVEMENT SERVICES

A bereavement follow-up service is provided as a component of the hospice program. Families' need continues after the death of one of their members. Bereavement counseling should be implemented as needed for at least fourteen to eighteen months following the patient's death. Grieving people often do not perceive the normality of their responses and behaviors. The bereavement team can be effective in the adjustment following the patient's death. Hospice encourages the expression of such grief as is consistent with the family's life style. Hospice staff recognize the value of social, religious, and ethnic practices in providing emotionally, socially, and ethnically acceptable outlets for such emotions. A hospice bereavement program provides a continuum of supportive and therapeutic services for the family, including formal and informal individual, family, and group treatment modalities.

Bereavement services are unique to hospice care; they are not provided anywhere else within the health care delivery system. Care of the family is continued after the death of the patient. Hospice work includes attention to needs of the bereaved, to assessment of needs of the bereaved, both before and after a death, and to the development of programs and resources to meet the needs of the bereaved. Hospice encourages the expression of grief, recognizes cultural variables in bereavement, and supports staff and family participation in meaningful funeral services and rituals (National Hospice Organization, 1982). This is one of the essential characteristics of a hospice program.

Persons experiencing grief are at a risk both physically and psychologically. If the strong emotions connected with grief are denied and socially condemned, maladaptive reactions may follow (Parkes, 1972).

A bereavement program includes three specific areas: individual support, group support and education, and the very important area of hospice staff support and education (Menapace, 1982). Programs to serve the bereaved need to offer various types of help to prevent the development of unnecessary pain and future physical and psychological problems.

Volunteers under the direction of a professional counselor can serve the needs of the bereaved family members and the hospice staff. The use of volunteers is further validated when one remembers that grief is a normal reaction, and support--not therapy--is indicated.

The bereavement counselor selects and properly trains the volunteers and coordinates the visitation to the bereaved family. The bereavement counselor will supply the necessary support and counseling, and referrals if necessary, for the bereaved family members that are experiencing abnormal or intense grief reactions.

The bereavement counselor organizes and facilitates the group support and education along with assistance from volunteers and guest speakers. The bereavement counselor also organizes and facilitates the hospice staff support group.

The term bereavement may be a difficult word to fully comprehend in today's society. The bereavement program can be named the Continuing Care Team.

The goals of the Continuing Care Team are:

1. To provide support and education about the grief process to the bereaved family. An emphasis is placed on the concept that grief is a normal response to the death of a loved one, and that this is a difficult process and requires hard work.

2. Visitation to the bereaved family is done informally by the direct care team and formally by the continuing care team.

3. The grieving process of the family members--and especially the primary care giver--is assessed by the team members.

4. High risk bereavers are closely monitored.

5. Communication between the continuing care team and the direct care team is emphasized.

6. The bereaved family is given information about the educational workshop.

7. The support given by the continuing care team is not intended to replace the primary or secondary support systems; instead, it is intended as an aid and a bridge to a rebuilding of life.

Thus, the bereavement program is part of the comprehensive hospice approach. Support and education are offered to the bereaved families. The message given to the families is that grief is normal; however, it is hard work and it takes time. The bereaved family members are not patients and normal grieving is not an illness. The members of the bereavement program will be there to help during this difficult time.

Now that we have thoroughly outlined the basic characteristics of hospice, we must examine in more detail its organization and administration.

REFERENCES

Brooks, Charles H., and Kathleen Smyth-Staruch. (1983). *Cost Savings Of Hospice Home Care To Third-Party Insurers.* Cleveland, OH: Hospice Council for Northern Ohio, Blue Cross of Northeast Ohio, and Case Western Reserve University.

Connecticut Hospice, Inc. (1984). *Pastoral Care Policies and Procedures.* Branford, CT.

Dailey, Ann A. (1984). *Children's Hospice International Newsletter* (Winter): 1-8.

Department of Health and Human Services, Health Care Financing Administration. (1983). Condition of Participation for Hospice Benefits under Medicare. *Federal Register.* December 16.

_____. (1984). Publication No.: HCFA 02154.

Frickey, Charles L. (1984). Reflections on Rural Hospice Care. *The American Journal of Hospice Care* 1(1):6-7.

Jenkins, Lowell, and Alicia S. Cook. (1981). The Rural Hospice: Integrating Formal and Informal Helping Systems. Paper presented at the Colorado Social Work Conference, Denver, Colorado.

Jivaff, L. (1979). *Home Care and The Quality of Life.* (E. Prichard, ed.). New York: Columbia Press.

Menapace, Nancy. (1982). *Bereavement Program.* Hospice of Pennsylvania, Inc. Typescript.

Munley, Anne. (1983). *The Hospice Alternative.* New York: Basic Books.

Munley, Anne, Cynthia S. Powers, and John B. Williamson. (1982). Humanizing Nursing Home Environments: The Relevance of Hospice Principles. *International Journal on Aging and Human Development* 15(4):263-283.

National Hospice Organization. (1982). *Standards of a Hospice Program of Care.* Arlington, VA.

Parkes, Colin M. (1972). *Bereavement.* New York: International Universities Press.

Pennsylvania Hospice Network. 1984. Handout, April 27th.

U. S. General Accounting Office. 1979. *Hospice Care--A Growing Concept in the United States.* HRD 79-50, March 6th.

Zimmerman, Jack. (1981). *Hospice: Complete Care for the Terminally Ill.* Baltimore-Munich: Urban and Schwarzenberg.

Chapter 3

Organization and Administration of Hospice Care

The evolution of hospice as a system and program of care, autonomously administered, has brought about the complexity of varied models of care. Since its beginning in the United States, hospice has been a grass roots movement with programs traditionally developed in communities in response to local need and in response to health care providers, and not in any one particular provider setting or type. Most new programs were modeled after their English counterpart incorporating the basic tenets of hospice care as outlined earlier in Chapter 2. The trend has been to locate hospices within already existing home care agencies, hospitals, and nursing facilities in order to achieve reimbursement mechanisms. The existence of third-party reimbursement appears to determine the general availability of hospice services. The recent hospice benefit under Medicare has provided an alternative for selected patients within a *small* number of hospices as discussed later in this chapter under *Seek Funding Sources*. Because hospice care is a nontraditional approach to organizing health care, community, and family resources to provide a total support structure for the terminally ill patient and family, several different models of hospice programs have evolved based upon the characteristics of the communities they serve.

In considering this dilemma of the number of hospice provider types, hospice advocates need to focus on the generic organizational principles which can be applied to all hospice models in order to assume continuity and coordination of care, quality care, and a viable program. Interplay between institutional and noninstitutional care is essential, particularly during the stages of the disease process when the patient's condition is changing rapidly. Short-term inpatient care is needed to assess changing medical needs and to provide respite for the family experiencing severe emotional and physical strain associated with a dying patient. However, most of the time noninstitutional services in the form of home care can be provided on a coordinated basis. An understanding of the importance of general management principles and concepts in administering a hospice program has been lacking. The limitations of current literature as to organizational strategies relative to quality hospice care is apparent. Therefore, it is timely to create sensitivity to and an awareness of the behavioral science approach to management of hospice programs. The reasons the findings of the behavioral science movement must be integrated into hospice management are many and varied. A basic climate of the hospice organization is sought by the creation of:

- open and free-flowing communication,

- increased productivity through concerted group effort,

- participative decision making,

- improved superior-subordinate relationships,

- integration and improvement of human and economic objectives,

- enriched job content and individual freedom as motivational factors.

Among a myriad of theories and writings, there are major philosophical and theoretical influences which must capture the imagination of hospice managers significantly more than others. Some notable theorists include: Douglas McGregor, Abraham Maslow, Frederick Herzberg, Rensis Likert, Chris Argyris, and Robert Blake with Jane Mouton (Rush, 1969). For a more detailed discussion of these particular theories, see pp. 71-72 in the section headed Staff Effectively.

Techniques and methods may be varied but they must be based on the characteristics of hospice care in order to reflect accurately correct hospice management. Organizational structure, management concepts and techniques, and administrative goals are not worth anything unless the implementation process is written and carried out to help the hospice patient/family attain the therapeutic goals for each problem.

Nevertheless, the approaches to management which stand out for hospice organizational development are those involving sensitivity training designed to impart increased understanding of one's own behavior, the behavior of others, and the impact of one's own behavior on others. Staff support sessions can provide an environment for this purpose. Any individual working within a hospice program must be aware of his or her own feelings concerning the death process in relation to self as well as others.

Blake and Mouton's Managerial Grid, designed to evaluate behavior in terms of managerial style and concern for people and production problems, provides a conceptual basis for personal and organizational assessment. Thoughtful attention to needs of people for satisfying relationships in hospice leads to a friendly, comfortable atmosphere and work tempo allowing staff to feel secure and good about themselves *and* hospice when giving care to patients. Work accomplishment comes from committed, caring staff. An interdependent staff who share common goals for the organization leads to relationships of trust and respect.

Psychological theory--in terms of understanding the behavior of people in the world of work and the implications for leadership--has been discussed at the Menninger Foundation Seminars (Rush, 1969). Jobs play an important role in employees' lives and one cannot separate the job positions from the people who perform them. Family members of staff in the provision of hospice services, give time and are also committed to the concept. A manager must believe in the importance of a mentally healthy hospice care team and recognize the effect that supervision has on attitudes, productivity, and the emotional stability of the employee. Educational seminars and coursework are useful for managers in their awareness of these factors, and contribute toward the achievement of these goals.*

OVERVIEW OF STRATEGIES AND PRACTICES

A discussion of managerial functions is basic to the success of any health care organization. Planning, organizing, staffing, directing, and controlling are important features of organization and administration. A manager's function can be considered a circle of action in which each component leads to the next. At different phases in the life of a hospice, one or another management function may be dominant. More recently the role of the professional hospice health care practitioner as manager is further reinforced by legal, regulatory, and accrediting agencies, a posture which many of the beginning hospice programs did not wish to undertake. However, the issue of survival has crept into the early philanthropic services. Indeed, hospice management cannot allow the hospice concept to become buried within the maze of the already existing health care delivery system. For this reason the classic management functions and their interrelationships are emphasized. Managers must monitor the organization's environment to anticipate change and bring about the adaptive responses required for the hospice program's survival.

In order for hospice administrators to achieve the objectives of the organization, key functions must be addressed. *Planning* involves identifying goals and objectives, stating premises and assumptions, and developing specific, detailed plans for hospice care. *Organization* follows: work must be broken down into components such as programs of education, home care, bereavement, volunteer, inpatient, outpatient, and adult day care. Next it is important to *group related work activities* and units. *Defining authority relationships* to establish management roles allows a basis for development of the organization chart and

---

* One example is a five-day course entitled, *Problem Solving Techniques for Modern Management*, offered within the graduate health services administration program at Marywood College's Department of Public Administration. In this course, Dr. Ann Marie Greco defines and develops managerial concepts, analytical techniques, and basic skills required of an administrator utilizing the dynamics of group problem-solving.

position descriptions. A critical function of a hospice manager which comes into focus next is that of *directing, actuating, and motivating*: a manager must be able to communicate objectives to members, lead members to objectives, train, supervise, and integrate the individual into the organization. Finally, a manager must be the *controlling or policing operation* of the organization, although a hospice supervisor seeks to create a positive climate so that the staff are motivated to conform, which will limit the amount of control that must be imposed. Still, staff must accept control mechanisms such as medical record audits, site visits, special reports, and time sheets (Liebler, Levine, and Dervitz, 1984).

Hospice programs have developed as a health care reform out of the concerns of professionals. These programs are a reaction against the runaway growth of technology in managing life-threatening and terminal illness at the expense of human dignity (Wald, Foster, and Wald, 1980). Individuals who share a common vision and set of values have come together to create a formal organization--hospice--for purposes that are consistent with and derived from their common values.

TEN COMMANDMENTS FOR STARTING A HOSPICE PROGRAM

Plan Reflectively

Planning, defined as the process of making decisions in the present to bring about an outcome in the future, is the most fundamental management action which logically precedes all other management functions (Levey and Loomba, 1973). Initially, the new hospice group must develop a statement of philosophy. The statement of philosophy or underlying purpose provides an overall frame of reference for organizational practice; it is the basis of the overall goals, objectives, policies, and derived plans. Currently, a "mission statement" is required as an overall goal for the hospice organization. Typically, the mission and philosophy statements developed for hospice programs are based upon national guidelines (National Hospice Organization, 1982; Department of Health and Human Services, 1983). The philosophy statement is critical to the hospice program since hospice evolved not as a place or institution but as a philosophy of care. Standard mission statements read as follows:

> Hospice, a community-based model of care, is a program of palliative and supportive services which provides physical, psychological, social, and spiritual care for terminally ill persons and their families. Services are provided by a medically supervised interdisciplinary team of professionals and volunteers. Hospice services are available in both home and in an inpatient setting; home care is provided on a part-time, intermittent, regularly scheduled, and around-the-clock basis. Bereavement services are available to the family. Admission to a hospice program of care is on the basis of patient and family need. Hospice provides a comprehensive

continuation of care utilizing an integration of appropriate services to eliminate duplication and fragmentation.
Hospice affirms life. Hospice exists to provide support and care for persons in the last phases of incurable disease so that they might live as fully and comfortably as possible. Hospice recognizes dying as a normal process whether or not resulting from disease. Hospice neither hastens nor postpones death. Hospice exists in the hope and belief that, through appropriate care and the promotion of a caring community sensitive to their needs, patients and families may be free to attain a degree of mental and spiritual preparation for death that is satisfactory to them.
Hospice is a community-based program of specialized health care which does not end when acute care is completed. Total patient care extends to the management of his dying and his death and extends even beyond, to his surviving family. Hospice teaches a new attitude toward dying and death, with the realization and conscious acceptance of dying and death as part of being born and part of the struggle of life. The concept of hospice is that the terminally ill should be allowed to die at home or in surroundings more home-like and congenial than the usual hospital setting.

In addition to reflecting the values of the immediate, specific group that formed the organization, a statement of philosophy may reflect, implicitly or explicitly, the values of the larger society.

Planning is facilitated when the mission statement and philosophy are formally stated. The need for planning stems from our changing external and internal environments and human limitations and concerns. In today's health care world, interdependencies abound. Planning is a dynamic, continuous activity that is influenced by all of the interacting elements related to the organization. Everyone involved in the program should take part in the planning process for the dual purpose of generating appropriate ideas and information and reducing resistance to future changes (White, 1981). A hospice group must not work alone since any plan affects others within the health care delivery system. When people work alone, without consulting others, their planning needs may be neglected at some cost to themselves but without directly affecting the flow of work to others. Hospice care plans must mesh with all disciplines and supportive services including related agency expectations and capabilities to sustain results achieved in the health care service. The overall transaction between systems must be carefully considered--inpatient, outpatient, home care, and community agencies--and planned in order to achieve coordination and quality results. Emphasis entails tailoring the hospice program to meet the needs of the individual local community, which can only be accomplished by knowing the influences--cultural, social, economic, political--in concert with a knowledge of the community profile and gaps in health care delivery. The importance of input from all segments surfaces immediately--the health care practitioners, educators, church leaders, business executives, other professionals, and the lay population.

In addition, another external factor which must be reviewed is the regional and state plan under the Health System Agency (HSA). This is a positive aspect simply because many organizations have found that strategic planning has been in their best interest. Plans help to anticipate events and avoid continual crises intervention, since a well-thought-out course of action specifies certain events that need to occur, when, where, and how they should occur, and who should insure their occurrence. Objectives, procedures, and evaluation criteria become clearer and more acceptable to all parties in the explication process involved in planning.

The objectives of the organization are equally important and are related closely to planning. Objectives specify a particular state of affairs that one intends to affect or change. For hospice programs, these objectives need to clarify that hospice care is a *nontraditional* way of organizing and delivering existing services including

- acute inpatient services
- subacute inpatient services
- outpatient services
- home health services
- patient education, counseling, and social services
- drug and rehabilitation therapies (Pryga and Bachover, 1983).

More specifically, hospice is *not* a place--as its historical definition might suggest--and it is *not* a particular type of service; it is a concept: care rather than cure. A distinguishing feature of hospice care is the goal of maximizing the quality of life for terminally ill patients.

An objective should fully declare the outcome of the effort: what one will do and how and why it will be done. An objective should result in action in pursuit of the declared intention (McCool and Brown, 1977). An example of beginning objectives for any hospice program might read as follows:

- To manage terminal illness in such a way that patients can live with their loved ones as they are dying, that their loved ones can go on living afterward with a minimum of problems, and that patients receive the best in medical and clinical interdisciplinary services available.

- To develop a patient care plan, including medical care, casework therapy, and nursing services, in order to improve the quality of life for 100 percent of the hospice patients and their families by helping them to share their feelings and problems related to living with a life-threatening illness.

- To make available pastoral counseling services in order to preserve the peace of mind of each patient as he relates to his own spiritual needs which will reassure and help the patient to offer his independence, dignity, and the human values he cherishes as he enters the final stage of his growth, the moment of death.

- To offer a comprehensive teaching and counseling program to patients and their families which will enable the patient to share more fully with his family his diagnosis, therapeutic plan, alternatives to that plan, anticipated side effects of medication, and the nature of all aspects of care.

- To provide day-to-day palliative and supportive care through professional and volunteer services for patients, as well as support for their families, and to focus this care on independence and involvement in decision making.

- To provide an educational mechanism for the community as to the availability and values of the hospice program, and to the role that community members may play in the fulfillment of its values.

- To manage, coordinate, and supplement rather than duplicate existing community services.

- To provide a process for coordinating hospice services with comprehensive medical and nursing services.

- To promote positive attitudes in acceptance of illness.

- To provide a therapeutic climate through use of an interdisciplinary team in order to ensure the ability of the family to follow through on the care plan.

- To provide additional source of in-service training for existing health care providers and to provide access to educational programs and seminars for local colleges and universities.

- To establish an additional resource to the existing health care services in the community.

- Without regard to color, race, religious creed, lifestyle, handicap, ancestry, national origin, union membership, age, or sex. (Prohibits discrimination).

These objectives will be translated into action when program development starts. Objectives add the dimension of quality, accuracy, and priorities to the mission statement and goals.

Changing national health goals and objectives acquire shifts in local and state resource allocation and altered health plans for new health care processes. The way in which a specific national or state policy affects a given local or specific organization's operations will vary according to circumstances and choices made locally. Hospice proponents need to structure their programs very carefully, for the greatest fear since the beginning of the hospice movement has been that the philosophy and concept might become *lost* in the system instead of *applied* to the existing system. According to Dooley (1982), the sad thing is that many hospices have compromised the ideals of hospice care in order to survive. Before more compromises further erode the hospice philosophy, the trade-offs should be carefully assessed through thoughtful organization and administration in order to ensure the movement's continuing integrity and survival.

Develop A Viable Organizational Structure

All organizations have a structure, and frequently it is written out as an organizational chart. However, a well-structured organization is no guarantee of services and no structure is sacrosanct. A structure that may work at one time might not work at a later time. It may give one an idea about authority, relationships, and distance, but it does not provide an in-depth understanding of power, personalities, or functions.

The organizational chart for hospice programs will vary according to the model of care. Hospital-based hospices will show up as a separate entity within a corporate structure whereas a community-based hospice will have a separate table of organization as shown in this example:

HOSPICE CORPORATE STRUCTURE

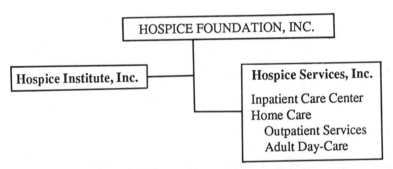

Hospice Foundation, Inc. functions as property holder for the other corporations and as a grantor of funding for educational and research proposals. The foundation may also assume the management responsibility via a contract to service and other programs. Hospice Services, Inc. provides direct services to program participants and acts as a base for education and research. Hospice Institute, Inc. acts as evaluator of proposed research and educational programs offered to Hospice Foundation for grants. The institute coordinates approved proposed programs with formal and continuing educational sources and conducts research into the outcomes.

A private corporation utilizes the planning components--mission statement and philosophy--and organizational components to establish articles of incorporation and by-laws in order to become legally incorporated (Inc.) by law.

Traditional issues which need to be considered in discussions of structure are span of control, division of labor, departmentalization, and delegation. The hospice care team is unique in that role blurring occurs in caregiving, an important deviation from the usual approach to delivery of services. Team members who perceive other members as having similar interests, knowledge, and goals often face conflict in the line of duty. Interdisciplinary health education is not presently a reality. Both nurses and social workers are seeking to expand their professional roles to include functions that traditionally belonged to the other's profession, and role overlap is inevitable. Conflict arises when members of the hospice care team intervene in patient and family care without earlier collaboration. According to Donovan (1984), paradoxically, conflict in teamwork can be minimized by more overlap of role functions in caring for terminally ill patients. The different skills and knowledge of nurses and social workers are needed in unison to solve the complex problems of the hospice patient and family. Different kinds of expertise are essential contributions to providing coordinated, comprehensive hospice services. The effective utilization of the expertise of each professional to solve these complex problems will enhance the quality of care. Working together in partnership while maintaining mutual respect for each other's knowledge and contributions will decrease conflict and allow freedom for achievement of professional realization.

Structure is not static; it is an important management tool to utilize in the quest for desired outcomes. It is sometimes imperative that an organization be restructured to recognize the particular talents of valuable people who act as catalysts for the development and maintenance of an effective organization (Goldsmith, 1981).

Finally, hospice leadership and management must be the responsibility of well-known community individuals who have a "handle" on the critical aspects of hospice--clinical services, referral sources, funding sources, expertise in financial and management implications, experiences with administrative concerns, the "bureaucratic maze," and especially, the needs of the people to be served.

Form Committees

The committee is paramount to the organizational process. Once the board of directors is appointed (when appropriate--such as in a separate agency model), the key committees must be selected from a cross-section of the community. Community support is essential in order for the hospice program to be viable. A professional advisory committee and a community advisory committee serve to meet the needs of the organization. Professional advisory committee members must be representative of the disciplines within the hospice care team and, in many ways, serve as ongoing peer reviewers. The responsibilities of this committee include recommending policy and monitoring all practices concerning services to patients and a quality assurance program for patient care.

In addition, the subcommittee--professional education/relations--arranges for ongoing education for physicians, nurses, social workers in health agencies and facilities, and staff in-service programs to train professionals for dealing with terminal patients and their families. This professional education/relations subcommittee supports information dissemination through publication, film, and other means to establish good working relations between hospice, health providers, and community clergy. The counseling subcommittee--composed of representatives from psychiatry, clergy, and social work--formulates policies and content of staff-delivered counseling to patients and their families. The public relations subcommittee is responsible for recommending policies necessary to facilitate an area-wide public relations program utilizing all available resources and opportunities and for evaluating and reporting results of such programs to the board and committee.

For broader input, the community advisory committee should be composed of businessmen, labor leaders, public relations representatives, consumers, legislative persons, fund raisers, bankers, representatives of industry, and lay persons whose purpose includes community relations, community education, fund raising, volunteer recruitment, legislative awareness, and development of a public relations program through newsletters and a speakers bureau.

Other subcommittees are then formed as needed for specific assignments; for example, an audit committee under the professional advisory committee is responsible for setting up criteria and standards for practice for each discipline whose members consist of both staff and committee representatives. When programs are added, such as an inpatient and outpatient component in the community and home care models, a subcommittee for inpatient care would be appointed to develop policies. A program evaluation committee is responsible for an overall policy and administrative review and a clinical record review to determine the extent to which they promote patient care that is appropriate, adequate, effective, and efficient.

Coordination of action and assessment of the overall organizational impact of a decision may be facilitated when these committees bring together a number of specialists for organized deliberation. Commitment and involvement from committees and board provide a broad framework for spreading the hospice gospel throughout the community. In fact, coordination and discussion among committee members and managers pave the way for acceptance of the programs in the community. Moreover, committees also serve as major communication networks to disseminate information, persuade members of the relevance of plans, and educate about changes and their implications. Hospice programs need flexibility which often comes from committee input. Regular meetings of the committees are held as needed but they do meet at least every other month and offer recommendations to the board of directors. Minutes of all meetings are kept to document activities. The hospice board of directors grants the committee certain authority and utilizes these committees to facilitate the decision-making process involved in a rapidly growing program.

In summary, hospice committees are created to fulfill various specific needs:

- to gain the advantage of group deliberation

- to offset decentralization and consolidate authority

- to counterbalance authority

- to provide representation of interest groups and the entire community

- to promote coordination and cooperation

- to train members (Liebler, Levine, and Dervitz, 1984).

Committee chairmen* may become members of the executive committee of the board if established through the by-laws of the organization. In a beginning organization their input is necessary and therefore their role on the executive committee may be critical to success. On the other hand, because of the necessity of frequent and immediate decisions, a large executive committee can be a detriment to the growth of a hospice program. In my own experience, I have found that committee chairmen can be just as effective as board members and not sit on the executive committee.

In the organization and administration of hospice, active committees are valuable to the manager as a mechanism for progress. Numerous activities can best be handled outside of formal board meetings. Committee activities allow directors of hospice programs more time to spend in managing care. Initially, committee membership should include those individuals representing disciplines who were involved in formulating beginning objectives for specific practice such as psychiatrist, clergy, bereavement counselor, nurses, social workers, and therapists.

Develop Programs

Although the impetus for starting a hospice program often comes from higher level expectations in a community, the flow of initiative can come from all levels within the organization and community. The proliferation of hospice care, no matter what the form, has taken place almost entirely within the voluntary sector of the health care system (Amenta, 1984). This brings forth critical questions: Who might logically contribute to the success of the hospice program? Who will

---

* According to strict parliamentarian interpretation, the proper term is chairman, with the titles of Madam Chairman or Mister Chairman used as specific indicators.

supply the input necessary for the success of hospice? How can hospice be well-coordinated with subsystems and adjoining systems in delivery of services? What professionals need to be involved initially? How can administration and staff ensure continuation of high quality care? Coordination needs seem to increase as the number and variety of professionals affected increases in the health care world. The hospice program provides a continuum of inpatient and home care services through an integrated administrative structure. Continuity implies enough administrative and staff integration to ensure continuation of the same high quality care when the patient moves from home to inpatient care or vice versa. It also implies the capacity to respond to patient/family needs whenever they arise.

Program adoption requires concurrence of those involved in developing objectives and investigating external influences such as environmental problems and constraints. However, developing hospices must not overlook their community's natural resources. Coordination among community agencies and groups is essential in order to provide the ideal interdisciplinary effect with the support of one's local consumers. Program design furnishes a base for development of policies and reflects the hospice characteristics.

The goals of the organization originate in the common vision and sense of mission embodied in the statement of purpose or the underlying philosophy. Goals reflect the general purpose of the hospice organization and provide the basis for subsequent management action including program design. As statements of long-range organizational intent and purpose, goals are ends toward which activity is directed. Goals, like statements of philosophy, may be found in the organization's charter, articles of incorporation, statement of mission, or introduction to the official by-laws. As with the statement of philosophy, the overall goals may not bear a specific label; they may be identified only through common understanding. Derivative plans are developed consistent with the hospice concept and philosophy.

Initial policies must be developed for the overall organization as guidelines for decision making. Policies state the required, prohibited, or suggested courses of action (Liebler, Levine, and Dervitz, 1984). Policies permit and require interpretation; therefore they are written in broad language for flexibility. Policies decide issues beforehand and limit actions so that situations that occur repeatedly are handled in the same way; this contributes to an atmosphere of stability. Policy statements are required for certification and they become part of the administrative manual. For example, in order to comply with the provisions of Title VI of the Civil Rights Act of 1964, Section 504 of the Rehabilitation Act of 1973, and the Age Discrimination Act of 1975, a nondiscrimination policy is required and reads as follows:

> It is the policy of Hospice to comply with the provisions of Title VI of the Civil Rights Act of 1964, Section 504 of the Rehabilitation Act of 1973 and the Age Discrimination Act of 1975, and all requirements imposed pursuant thereto, to the end

that *no* person shall, on the basis of age, race, color, national origin, religion and or handicap be excluded from access to and receipt of services, be excluded from participation in, be denied benefit of, or otherwise be subjected to discrimination in the provision of any care or service, programs or activities.

This nondiscriminatory policy of Hospice applies to patients/families, physicians, and all responsible employees. Under no circumstances will the application of this policy result in patient segregation or resegregation for reasons of age, race, color, national origin, religion and/or handicap. Hospice is an affirmative action/equal opportunity employer.

Other policies which may be required initially are acceptance of patient/family care policies, interdisciplinary group policy, patient care policies, continuation of patient care policies, patient care coverage and coordination policy, medical record policies, personnel policies, and patient grievance procedure. Appendix A, B, and C are samples of policy. These appendices are on pp. 239-247.

From policy formulation a procedure manual must be developed to include areas such as patient care protocols. Procedures are developed to ensure uniformity of practice for quality services. The newer patient care protocols developed for hospice care involve symptom management and pain control. Appendix D on pp. 249-256 gives an example of nursing procedures required for care to hospice patients.

Program components which require development for any hospice program of care, in specific order, are:

1. Education

2. Volunteers

3. Home Care

4. Inpatient Care

5. Bereavement

6. Outpatient Care

Adult Day Care adds continuity to hospice services and will be discussed further in Chapter Eleven.

Education. Education of professionals in the community is of paramount importance prior to starting a hospice program of care. The physician, as a key member of the team and a prime referral source, must be alert to the effects which the hospice philosophy of care has on the terminally ill patient and family. Working with the local medical society on a jointly-sponsored seminar to which a nationally known and respected physician is invited to speak is a first step in setting up any hospice program. In 1978, during the planning stages of Hospice of Pa., Inc. a physician from St. Lukes in New York spoke to the members of the local medical society. A question was asked: How does hospice care differ from our traditional care to patients? One slide answered this question: it showed the physician sitting on a chair at the patient's bedside early in the morning holding the patient's hand and looking into her face as he interviewed her regarding her pain and the effects of the pain medication during the night which was being given every four hours around the clock. The physician sat and interviewed the patient for as long as necessary to gather information as to the type, severity, and location of the pain. More and more physicians have an interest in and are becoming involved in hospice, especially the family practitioner and the oncologist. Physicians need to spend as much time as possible with their patients during their final days and hours. By becoming more familiar with the clinical and emotional signs of impending death, physicians can contribute a great deal of information for final decision making (Ufema, 1984).

Concurrently in-service education programs should be conducted within the local hospitals, nursing homes, and other health organizations for nurses, social workers, therapists, and other interested members of the health care team. Once the health care professionals in the community are educated as to hospice care, presentations need to be scheduled with the myriad of community groups such as service clubs, church groups, schools, and other community organizations. Ongoing community presentations should be scheduled and publicized as much as possible.

Monthly in-service programs for hospice care staff planned on an annual basis are effective in improving the level of expertise for individual staff members. Funds should be allocated in the hospice budget for staff to attend specialized programs as provided for in education policies discussed earlier in Chapter 2. Through a hospice continuing education program, staff members develop a deeper appreciation of their role as a member of the team.

Educational procedures must be carefully developed in any hospice program based on certain priorities and objectives. The size and composition of the group may need thoughtful deliberation to determine appropriate sessions. One example is staff support sessions which are more beneficial when held for the different staff groups--office support, caregivers, various disciplines, supervisors, administrators. A staff-designated counselor reassures employees that the organization is providing efforts to support them as members of the hospice team. In addition, open communication becomes an element of hospice, and counseling can be used to maintain constructive attitudes. Good morale is critical to hospice managers. Staff orientation, "on-the-job" training, and educational programs become key elements of personnel management in hospice care.

Program evaluation of the educational component of hospice allows effectiveness to be measured. Aside from testing before and after an educational session for knowledge measures, observation for improved methods of practice and behavioral changes relate the true value of educational programs in hospice.

Volunteers. Most hospices started through the efforts of medical care professional volunteers who recognized that certain needs of the terminally ill were not being met in the community. These professionals gave their time and expertise to draft a program which included establishing by-laws, incorporating, attaining nonprofit status, selecting a board of directors, and raising funds. Volunteers are the backbone of hospice care giving (Bunn, 1984). As discussed in Chapter 1 under economic influences, volunteer services are required under the new hospice benefit under Medicare. In order to be a certified hospice, five percent of the total patient care hours must be provided by volunteers. In addition to direct service to patient and family, volunteer services include participation on a speaker's bureau for community education, office support, and fund raising. Volunteers have made it possible for hospice programs to expand and provide a comprehensive supportive service to the community.

Volunteer training sessions vary among hospices but include a comprehensive educational process with sharing of experiences. Topics may include:

- History and Philosophy of Hospice

- The Spiritual Dimension of Hospice

- Dynamics of Dying

- Communication and Creative Listening Skills

- Coping Mechanisms

- Current Theory and Methods in Diagnosis and Treatment of Cancer

- Family and a Unit of Care

- The Bereavement Process

- Developing Sensitivity in Patient Care

- The Hospice Care Team

- Dealing with Anger and Resistance with Family In Crises

- Administrative Issues

The types of volunteer services are vast as identified in Chapter 2. Respite care is a concern of all models; the community-based sites are able to provide it more than the others. There is wide recognition of the need for respite for families. It is understood that respite care is conducive to cost-effectiveness since it enables patients to be cared for longer in the home setting, thereby avoiding the cost of expensive hospitalization. Respite includes anything from the volunteer staying for a time, to the patient being an inpatient for a few days to provide the family with a time to rest. Transportation, errand services--such as grocery and drug store shopping, homemaking services--such as meal preparation and household chores, and volunteer patient care services--such as putting the patient to bed are valuable hospice services.

In some models, the director of volunteer services is responsible for the management of the volunteer department. The director encourages and cooperates with other staff and volunteers to (1) ensure that volunteers are utilized as an integral component of the Hospice program; (2) set goals and objectives for volunteer services; (3) plan policies and procedures; (4) identify job descriptions; (5) select and assign volunteers with consideration for the skills, knowledge, and motivation of the individual and the goals of hospice; (6) provide for the orientation of new volunteers; (7) provide guidance during the early stage of work and ongoing inservice education; (8) structure the organization to include the supervision and support of volunteer personnel; (9) provide for individual job performance evaluation, growth, and mobility; and (10) provide for volunteer participation in planning and evaluation of the program.

Volunteers participate in an individualized orientation course planned by the director of volunteer services based on the applicant's education, experience, and skills in relation to the assignment.

The volunteer director must be aware of the importance of recruiting volunteers with special skills instead of relying on volunteers who may bring their own problems into the situation (Jaffe, 1981). Methods of recruitment include notices in church bulletins and contact with church groups, public speaking by volunteers including board and committee members, and staff and press coverage in newspapers and local publications. According to volunteer directors some recruitment problems have surfaced. Often, a bereaved family member will seek a volunteer role before the bereavement process is completed; this can create a hardship for patient and volunteer alike. For this reason, most hospice volunteer programs mandate a waiting period of six months to a year after any major loss of a family member. If enough time is allowed, many of these volunteers become excellent hospice workers and bring a special sensitivity to their volunteer duties.

Volunteer recruitment, therefore, requires a major effort by the director/coordinator of volunteers through the media, community presentations, word-of-mouth, church and synagogue bulletins and announcements, posters, and special community days, for example, career day, health day.

The volunteer coordinator directs all recruitment, education, and training as well as assignments. In some hospices, an assistant volunteer coordinator is required to assure a smooth operation and quality services. Rules and procedures are incorporated into a volunteer handbook. Proper administration of a hospice volunteer program is clearly important to quality of patient/family care.

Home Care. The organization and administration of the home care component is best served by a community-based model of direct care. This requires the hospice to become a certified home care agency. While some states require certificate of need for home care, others do not, allowing the hospice to receive reimbursement through the certification process. Three reasons stand out in favor of this whenever possible:

- Central administration with professional management responsibility

- Control and coordination

- Provision of home care services only to hospice patients

The traditional home health agency which expands into a hospice program provides care either through an identified hospice team with an oncology nurse or as a specialty service of all staff to identified hospice patients. These programs have similar informal arrangements for inpatient care. This provider type now represents about 18 percent of the providers in the country (McCann, 1983).

In contrast, most hospital-based hospice programs have contractual arrangements with existing traditional home care agencies which research shows limits coordination and decreases quality control.

The recent federal legislation mandates that 80 percent of the care be provided in the home. According to the Government Accounting Office report in 1979, about half of the hospice services in the nation were home care programs. In view of these statistics, management expertise needs to focus on home care organization and development. As discussed earlier, an added dimension which some hospice home care programs find effective is a supportive program of private duty care administered by the hospice organization. Its purpose is to maintain family unity and independent living in times of illness and other stressful situations, to provide additional care to those patients who wish to remain in the home, and to permit family members and/or caregivers more time for themselves. Supportive care services usually include nursing, nursing assistants, homemakers, and companions. The individuals who provide services require special hospice training, are employed by hospice, and become members of the hospice care team.

Inpatient Services. Hospital-based hospice programs provide inpatient services either in a discrete unit or a scattered bed program. Research conducted by this author showed that better quality of care is provided in a discrete unit for identified hospice patients. There appears to be less overlapping of lines of authority. In a scattered bed situation team members provide consultation services to hospice patients wherever they are in the hospital. Regular staff deliver the services to patients. Staff training throughout the hospital on hospice patient care protocol becomes a vast undertaking due to staff turnover and absenteeism. Hospital-based hospice comprise about 40 percent of the known providers (McCann, 1983). Hospice units and programs are organized and staffed differently than medical/surgical units in the average hospital. They are usually governed by different policies and procedures. There are inherent problems in providing inpatient hospice care in acute-care institutions, because the philosophies underlying the two kinds of care are diametrically opposed. The goals of today's acute-care hospital are sophisticated curative care and maintenance of life; the goal of the hospice is good palliative care and maintenance of dignity (McNulty and Holderby, 1983). Because of such different philosophies of care there are usually different policies and procedures governing hospice units or programs. The patient and family is the unit of care. The goal is to make it possible for them to be together as much as possible, to share the last few precious moments together. Relaxing the visiting hours and rules is one way of doing this which may cause problems in an acute-care hospital.

Long-term care based hospice programs are most often found in skilled nursing facilities and involve one to three identified beds. Organizationally, hospice care may, perhaps, fit more comfortably in a nursing home, where the focus is on rehabilitation or custodial care rather than cure. The average nursing home is not prepared to provide the interdisciplinary team of caregivers or enough volunteers to meet the goals of good hospice care. Nevertheless, skilled nursing beds appear to be a more appropriate level of care.

Due to economic constraints freestanding hospices have not been practical as demonstrated in this author's research project.

Considering all inpatient settings discussed here, it seems ironic that the model conducive to quality of care based on the organizational structure is the skilled care facility, a direction hospices traditionally have not pursued. Home care hospices having formal arrangements with hospitals and nursing homes for inpatient care based on patient and family needs seems a valid and logical administrative approach to hospice care. A trend toward hospital scattered-bed approach rather than discrete units is apparently due to the recent reimbursement process.

Bereavement. The degree of sophistication varies in the bereavement program from site to site and among models. A pattern has emerged to use volunteers for bereavement counseling due to cost factors and lack of reimbursement from third parties for bereavement counseling. This too explains the reasons for the variations which are due to limited time, staffing, and lack of funding. Some programs use volunteers or paid staff who were previously unknown to the family to provide bereavement services. The literature confirms the philosophy that a new person can be a more helpful listener than someone who might have previously established biases about the family members and family dynamics. Generally, the attitude toward bereavement is that grieving is normal though there are a few persons who really need professional (psychiatric) intervention; most do well with some support from hospice. Some bereaved do well with no intervention at all. Therefore, some programs are now developing ways to identify those who are at special psychological risk during bereavement so these individuals find appropriate care. Adult block grant funds are now available in some communities for counseling to eligible clients; this includes hospice bereavement counseling. Also the new outpatient reimbursement program, Comprehensive Outpatient Rehabilitation Facility (CORF), discussed later in this chapter provides a funding source for counseling, which could, in fact, begin to set a pattern for these services on the basis of the funding resource alone. Currently, bereavement counseling is required by federal legislation under the hospice Medicare benefit.

In many hospital-based model programs, there are regularly scheduled socials or coffees where the bereaved come and find the needed support from one another. Other inpatient programs invite their families to a monthly bereavement group session. The patient care coordinator writes bereavement notes regularly from "friends at hospice" inviting families to attend the bereavement group and to feel free to call if they need any help.

A bereavement brochure is effective to remind families of hospice services. Staff members or volunteers attend the wake or funeral and a sympathy card is sent within three days. Since hospice programs are finding it necessary to carry out the bereavement program totally through volunteer efforts, it is always best to have a paid staff professional as a director/coordinator.

Bereavement counseling is made available to the hospice patient and family prior to death and continues as needed for at least fourteen to eighteen months following the patient's death. Included in bereavement services are home visits as needed, support groups, and assistance in necessary life adjustments.

Some bereavement programs are based on needs and priorities to high-risk bereavement families because of limited staffing and the cost of such services which are not covered under third-party reimbursement. Prior to the death of the patient, the hospice personnel conduct a prebereavement assessment to determine those who are highly stressed or emotional and who may require additional support during the bereavement process. Hospice personnel contact all individuals primarily responsible for the patient prior to death to explain the supportive services which are available in the bereavement program. No contact is made after the death of the patient if the primary individual indicated that they do not wish to be contacted. Immediately following the death of the patient, the nurse specialist or social worker contacts the primary individual to assist the family with finances, will, insurance, and funeral arrangements. Subsequent phone calls and/or visits are made as needed but at least in two weeks, one month, three months, six months, and one year from the date of death; then more calls are made as needed. The bereavement assessment process limits the number of families in the bereavement program allowing a more comprehensive approach in relation to staff and time constraints.

The bereavement program development, training, and coordination is mainly the responsibility of the bereavement coordinator/director. However, as discussed, the nurse, social worker, other team members and volunteers help make up the bereavement teams. The general procedure upon the demise of the patient is a visit to the home of the family and the funeral home. Further, this person attends the funeral itself and assists by keeping in close contact with the bereaved for an ensuing eighteen-month period. The hospice team also acts as a consultant to any family medical problems that may arise following the loss of a loved one.

This description of the variations and ongoing changes in bereavement programs demonstrates the focus for the proper administration and implementation of this program for maximum effectiveness.

Bereavement program development, therefore, does require a bereavement counselor as the program coordinator in order to provide the expertise required for this sensitive program. The goal is to help the bereaved family experience and work through their grief. The bereavement counselor should have a master's degree with major course work in psychology, counseling and health-related areas with two years of clinical work experience. This person could be a nurse or social worker. The bereavement counselor is responsible for the necessary training program of the continuing care team where both cognitive and experiential learning is addressed. An effort is made to develop a cohesive team effort. Members of the continuing care team include a staff psychiatric consultant, bereavement counselor, and volunteers.

Existing bereavement programs include approximately twenty-four hours of training. Areas addressed are:

- information about the hospice concept

- information concerning the holistic approach to caregiving

- basic listening and attending skills

- current concepts about dying, death, and bereavement

- family dynamics that include the general systems approach

- communication skills

- an in-depth understanding of the bereavement program and the technical information about procedures and office routine.

It is necessary to have an accessible resource information area. Included in Appendix E on pp. 257-259 are annotated bibliographies of selected material. Three very readable, nontextbooks should be made available for the use of the staff and bereaved family members. The titles are: *How to Survive the Loss of a Love* (Bloomfield), *Someone You Love is Dying: A Guide for Helping and Coping* (Shepard), and *The Gift of Grief* (Tanner). See Appendix E (Menapace, 1982). Additional resource material needs can be better determined after program experience is gained. These requests will have to be balanced with the availability of funds.

Another excellent source of material is the U.S. Government; many publications are available for free or a nominal fee. Duplications of journal articles can also be made available for a nominal fee. The resource material would be for the benefit of the hospice staff, as well as the bereaved families. Two excellent resources which include forms used in a bereavement program are *Bereavement Care Manual*, written and compiled by Marcia Lattanzi and Diane Coffelt, and *Bereavement: A Guide for Training*, by Riverside Hospice.

Sample procedures which are very specific and necessary for a quality bereavement program are shown in Appendix F on pp. 261-269. A contract is recommended for the continuing care team; an example is displayed in Appendix G. Components of a brochure on the Continuing Care Team Program for family members is shown in Appendix H on pp. 273-274.

A memorial service and reception for families of deceased patients provides an excellent spiritual and social environment during holidays.

Finally, a critical aspect of the services of any bereavement program is the educational process. The educational workshop is the basis for organizing the bereavement component of any hospice program.

Freud stated in his work *Mourning and Melancholia* (1907/1959) that to be made aware of why one is anxious and to understand the origin of anxiety will in itself lessen the anxiety. For this reason an educational workshop is chosen instead of an ongoing bereavement person's group. The experience of other hospice bereavement programs that have successfully used the educational workshop model have found the bereaved person's support group less satisfying. However, as the program becomes established a support group may prove to be a viable option. Some hospice programs have found the bereavement support group to be more successful after the educational process is completed. The workshop model recommended is the one outlined by the Riverside Hospice, *Bereavement: A Guide for Training*. (See *Appendix E*, page 258). The guide presents detailed information for a program that includes six workshops. Reference material is also provided along with practical suggestions for organizing the workshops. The workshop can be organized and facilitated by the bereavement counselor or with assistance from volunteers and guest speakers. The topics suggested for the workshop are:

- Loss and Grief
- Family Changes
- Single Parents
- Remembering
- Intimacy
- A New Life

The workshop topics will be responsive to the needs of each particular group. An additional session can be added if the group so desires.

It is suggested that groups be by age. A heterogenic group for below age fifty-five and a group for over age fifty-five is suggested. It would be difficult for a young bereaved person to relate to the needs of an elderly bereaved person and vice versa.

The guide suggests that the workshop only be offered to bereaved individuals six months after the death of their loved one. However, a bereaved individual can use this information and support after one month of bereavement.

The first group would be made up of individuals whose loved ones were a part of the hospice program. An invitation would be issued to all families that have had a death within the last eighteen months. One week after mailing the invitations a telephone call from the hospice office would be made. At this time any questions could be answered and arrangements made for the person to attend the workshop.

The guide also suggests that from six to eighteen persons be included in each workshop. However, based on the author's experience, any number over fifteen would be counterproductive. Volunteers and staff members may be included as further support for the bereaved individuals.

An inviting and comfortable room is necessary for the proper atmosphere in the workshop. Arrangements are necessary to provide a room that meets these criteria and is easily accessible to the workshop members.

Direct caregivers support group. Research has shown that caregivers are greatly affected by the death of their patients. To facilitate a group that will give support, empathy, and feedback to the direct care team a monthly support group is recommended.

The bereavement counselor organizes and facilitates the support group. The goals of the group are:

- Support
- Empathy
- Feedback
- Information
- Greater self-awareness
- Greater self-understanding

Future programs. The philosophy of hospice has been to develop programs slowly and carefully. To insure the success of the bereavement program the same careful approach should be taken.

The educational workshop for the bereaved appears to be a good starting point. As volunteers are trained and material is assembled the visitation program can be put into action.

Programs to be considered for future development might include:

• A bereaved person's group

• A crisis intervention training program for hospital personnel

• A training program for community agencies and religious organizations

• A bereaved parent's group

• A multifamily group workshop

These programs can be refined to meet the specific needs of each hospice program.

Outpatient Services. As of December 15, 1982 Comprehensive Outpatient Rehabilitation Facility (CORF) services under Medicare Part B were authorized under the Omnibus Reconciliation Act of 1980 (Department of Health and Human Services, 1982). Essentially, what CORF means is that by using many of the same services an agency may currently have in place, outpatient services can be established so that patients come to hospice to receive services as well as the home care staff going to them to provide services. Under the regulations, thirteen items and services are covered as CORF services: (1) physician services; (2) physical therapy; (3) occupational therapy; (4) speech-language pathology; (5) respiratory services; (6) prosthetic devices; (7) orthotic devices; (8) social services; (9) psychological services; (10) nursing care; (11) drugs and biologicals; (12) supplies, appliances, and equipment; and (13) home environment evaluation.

To receive medicare certification as a CORF, a hospice must comply with state and local laws; meet specified conditions pertaining to its governing body and administration; provide a coordinated rehabilitation program that includes at least physicians' services, physical therapy, and social or psychological services furnished by staff that meet specified qualifications; maintain clinical records on all patients; provide a physical environment that protects the health and safety of patients, personnel, and the public; have written procedures for handling of patients, personnel records, and the public in disaster situations; and have, in effect, a written utilization review plan to assess the need for services and promote the most efficient use of the services furnished by the facility. Major sources of information needed for the governing body and administration are:

• Articles of incorporation, bylaws, policy statements, and so on

- Minutes of governing body, staff, and patient care policy meetings

- Organization chart showing administrative framework

- Personnel records: job descriptions and personnel qualifications

- Institutional budget plan

- Management contracts

- Patient care policies

- Clinical records

A group of professional personnel is required. CORFs permit numerous services traditionally housed within hospitals to be strategically relocated in close proximity to the patient base. CORFs provide hospice a continuum of care by taking over services that do not require an expensive structure. Hospice patients covered under Medicare Part B can receive social, psychological, and other covered services as outpatients under CORF when home care or institutional care is not appropriate and in an atmosphere conducive to each service, such as counseling for readjustment therapy, physical therapy for pain and symptom management, and occupational therapy, to enable patients to maximize that independent state of being and living in the areas of self, work, and play.

Staff Effectively

Certain people need the excitement of working in young and developing programs, while others prefer to work in the older, more established programs. What is needed in all hospice programs is a group of hardy people who can stand up to the pressures of a medical staff that is likely to be less than enthusiastic. Hospice needs people who are motivated by challenge, responsibility, autonomy, and recognition more than financial or job security.

A concern about the program's existence in ten years should be as important as the excitement inherent in starting a new program. Continual changes may be required to keep that first team interested.

Managers must carefully examine not only the attitudes but also the behavior of the staff. Personal characteristics needed for personnel to be effective in hospice care and development include:

- Assertiveness based on a sense of being centered/grounded in a nourishing source of personal energy.

- Ability to operate productively without traditional role constraints.

- Ability to function under stress, to make decisions alone, and accept responsibility for them.

- Awareness of self with the ability and willingness to probe and monitor motivations and feelings.

- Openness to learning, growing, and changing as both work with patients and personal experience within the staff open greater understanding of self and hospice work.

- Sensitivity, intuition, and feeling qualities in marked degree.

- Recognition of death as a natural life experience.

- Recognition that hospice patients need support rather than traditional therapy.

Hospice directors must seek staff that fit the organization, yet be aware of the basic needs of individuals. Theories of motivation are applicable in hospice. The art of motivating is built on this recognition of human need. Maslow's (1954) theory of motivation is predicated on the premise that every action is motivated by an unsatisfied need. Once a need has been satisfied, another level of need is no longer a motivator. Maslow's hierarchy of needs consist of the following scale (from most basic need to higher level, self-actualizing needs):

- Physiological needs (food, water, air)

- Safety and security (order and stability)

- Belonging and social activity (a place in a group)

- Esteem and status (desire for acceptance, prestige)

- Self-fulfillment (full use of talents, self-actualization)

Herzberg, Mausner, and Snyderman (1959) approached the theory of motivation by identifying two factors that are operative in motivation: satisfiers and dissatisfiers. Examples of satisfiers as identified by Herzberg are opportunity for advancement and promotion, greater responsibility, opportunity for growth, and interesting work. His concept of motivators tends to parallel Maslow's higher needs levels--those of esteem and status and self-fulfillment as verbalized by hospice staff.

McGregor's (1960) view Applying Hospice organization is best served by Theory Y, wherein the manager assumes that work is as natural as rest or play; that the average worker, under the right conditions, seeks to accept responsibility; and that workers will exercise self-direction and self-control in the service of objectives to which they are committed. This is in opposition to his Theory X manager who feels employees dislike work, avoid work, have little ambition, and want security above all else.

Linked to Theory Y and Hospice is Theory Z which emphasizes long-range planning, consensus decision making, participative management, and strong, mutual worker employee loyalty. The five principles underlying Theory Z are:

(1) the need for goals; (2) positive and negative reinforcement; (3) correction of errors; (4) feedback systems; and (5) goal revisions (Zangwill, 1976). Group decision making and quality circles to foster worker involvement in decisions and control processes are elements of Theory Z (Ouchi, 1981), a contemporary approach to management and motivation which are important to hospice workers. The hospice care team becomes involved with critical decisions regarding patient and family care plans. Hospice with its small organizational size decreases barriers to communication. Supervisors of hospice care must motivate the team members and assist in the adaptation of the individual to the organizational demands. Individuals must "fit" into the organizational framework. There is a close tie between the motivation/adaptation activities and the controlling function of the manager. Hospice staff members who fit the organization and who value an assigned role are likely to be motivated more easily. In turn, the need to control activity, for example, through disciplinary action, is reduced (Rush, 1969).

Argyris (1957) argues that the individual's and the organization's objectives can be meshed. His theme of "job enlargement" is inherent in hospice practice. Job content can expand to include a wider range of tasks and to broaden the worker's control over his task. This calls for a program design to fit an individual's particular set of interests and skills to the organization's objectives. Implicit in job enlargement is interchange of tasks among hospice members to enhance the members' knowledge of each other's job and to gain more flexibility in meeting the hospice group's production objectives. Certainly a desired part of this interchange is the enrichment of the group's participation, interaction, and cohesiveness. Argyris's integration of the individual and the organization exemplifies a large segment of contemporary behavioral science's search for improved organizational effectiveness and optimized human motivation. Argyris discusses the dichotomy of individual needs and organizational needs in his research and writings. McGregor (1960) felt that organizations can frustrate human beings in the realization of their needs. Argyris (1964) agrees with this point, but he carries the argument a step further and posits that organizations may be the source and cause of human problems.

The nature of hospice care brings the element of stress to the forefront. People who are stressed must be managed carefully so that they are not additionally burdened. Staff support meetings are crucial in this regard. Much literature has been written on stress and burnout. In hospice, an alert supervisor must always be aware of the varied levels of stress and counter the causative elements through conferences, a social time, or even respite for the staff person. Each staff member must be trained to anticipate a level of saturation and react accordingly. Energies of hospice staff are high; therefore, they must be channeled constructively. Perception as a team player is a natural and essential aspect of the hospice care team. Putting in long hours requires a large amount of sheer physical energy, even though some time is spent in social rituals--like reading, informal conversation, discussion of newspaper articles and experiences, and taking coffee breaks. These rituals forge social bonds among hospice staff that make real managerial work--that is, group work of various formats--possible. One must participate in the rituals to be considered effective in caring for hospice patients and families. The interdisciplinary (IDG) team concept is most important to hospice care. Closeness of the work team, its homogeneity in hospice, and good morale have a positive effect on job satisfaction.

At the heart of a hospice program are regular meetings of team members to discuss and consider the needs of each individual patient. Each patient is discussed in detail so that the team members will know everything that is going on and thus make sure that what each says or does fits in with the total pattern and plan. Decisions are made as to which member of the team will ask which questions so that they do not duplicate one another's conversation. At the team meetings, the hospice staff is discussed as well to clarify particular needs and possible methods of assistance. Such regular discussions also keep members of the hospice team alerted to possible conflicts, so that tensions can be resolved before they become serious. Team meetings also serve to build the relationship among members of the hospice group themselves, so that they can better support one another. They talk things through, plan parties and celebrations together, seek to develop a philosophy of teamwork, and are alert to call on the assistance of a psychiatrist if there is a "blow-up."

Fundamental to the team approach is the concept that no one person has all the answers and that total care is made easier by a variety of personnel, with a variety of resources, working together. Such a team approach, however, is not an easy task, and members must resolve to break down interprofessional rivalries and set aside defensive attitudes. Communication is essential and requires both time and effort. Good communication is not only verbal--through regular meetings--but also must be written; careful records, which can be shared, must be kept. Through coordinated records of physicians, nurses, social workers, and others, the story of each patient unfolds so as to involve all members of the team. A basic step is Assessment--recognition that each family and patient are unique. Members of the hospice team have different personalities also. Each person has his or her own ideas about methods of work; the points of view may not always be initially in harmony. Early collaboration helps to define the role of each team member. The team and administrator must be in agreement about the job description of each team member. The tasks and roles of *each* member of the team are important. The hospice team has stated the following as its goals:

- To assist patients into a state where they experience relief from distressing symptoms, pain, and fear of pain.

- To achieve objective signs in patient indicating feelings of peace and security.

- To review patients weekly in team conferences to determine if goals of hospice care are appropriate.

- To ensure that patients experience increased contact with staff and volunteers as death approaches if they want and need it.

- To give patients and family the opportunity to draw closer together as death approaches.

- To support families in the bereavement process.

- To educate and assist staff in developing an awareness of their own response to death.

- To offer the staff the support of the hospice team and hospice committee as they work with the dying.

- To develop and maintain a program of continuing education and research for hospital staff.

- To provide staff who can support the patient and family through the grief and bereavement process.

The interdisciplinary (IDG) team meets regularly (daily or as needed) both formally and informally to discuss patient care, offer support to each other, and handle any administrative problems. These meetings also handle any stress factors encountered by team. In addition, staff support meetings are held monthly and conducted by the RN coordinators. Communications are carried out by telephone between meetings as needed.

Staff selection and staffing patterns are the key elements in providing a successful program. Hasty staff selection may result in recruitment of professionals who lack a basic understanding of the hospice concept. They also may lack the warmth, insight, and attitudes necessary to implement the hospice approach to care of the dying. Hospice workers are not made, they are born. Just as hospice is not for *every* patient and family, hospice is also not the type of work for every professional. Hospice staff need a special loving attitude by caring, compassionate, and sensitive professionals. Such a person needs a considerable amount of patience, awareness of one's own values and beliefs toward death, and expertise in the care of the dying (Rodek and Jacob, 1983).

Group and individual interviews of prospective staff by the person responsible for hospice services have been found helpful. Also several prospective staff may be interviewed by supervisory members of the IDG team. Interviewers should be trained in communication skills and interviewing techniques. In addition, if a prospective staff member needs further screening, the staff support counselor plans an interview in the person's home. The author's experience in utilizing this process has been most rewarding with very effective results for hospice staffing. Staff orientation and ongoing in-service education must be done well. Because of the nature of hospice care, there is usually a higher staff/volunteer to patient ratio with more care being given by volunteers than in the traditional programs. An effective staffing method to determine whether a new hospice care member "fits" into the hospice family is to start everyone on a part-time basis with one patient and family assignment at a time. This method of staffing gives both the individual and hospice supervisors time to observe each other and work together. If the individual is the sensitive person needed on the team and demonstrates excellent performance, then the person can be assigned on a full-time basis. This evaluation period is critical and necessary. This method of assignment also provides continuity.

The same hospice care team members care for the patient and family during their stay with the program to assure continuity of care. A natural back-up team develops within the overall team by each individual professional for their assigned patients and families. Also certain professionals and support team members function better if hospice remains a part-time employment for them along with a position in a conventional or educational setting. This reduces stress and gives an outlet for channeling their curative needs.

The role of the physician will be discussed later under the heading Establish Referral Sources. Family members are often the primary caregivers in hospice which means that the approach of hospice caregivers is often more instructive as a coordinator of care. The medical caregivers do not possess the control they enjoy in more traditional settings.

Finally, hospice administrators and caregivers must select a mentor. A mentor provides one with visibility and opportunities to showcase abilities and to make connections with those of higher status. The whole meaning of mentoring which embodies the concepts of collegiality and networking is workable both on an individual and organizational level. Developed hospice programs can work with new programs through guidance, teaching and helping the new hospice avoid pitfalls. An individual mentor can be a prestigious person with many experiences and special expertise, a colleague who has advanced in the profession and served the people either inside or outside the hospice--a teacher, a "living example of excellence whom one can respect." A mentor is a person one selects for assistance in meeting personal goals and in the case of the organization, organizational goals.

Productivity is achieved through quality circles and feedback sessions. Quality circles are trained, organized, structured groups who identify problems, find causes of the problems, develop solutions and present a proposal to management for approval and implementation. According to Drucker (1974), management must address the future, mold it, and balance short-range and long-range goals.

Seek Funding Sources

Most hospice models have utilized the traditional reimbursement sources for revenues in order to provide an ongoing funding mechanism for a continuing program. When starting a hospice program, third-party reimbursement is a critical factor. Grant awards are welcomed for program development but should not be the only beginning source of income. The reason for this is demonstrated by three programs originally funded under National Cancer Institute for three years. After that time, alternatives were necessary for continued services. The lack of third-party reimbursement for hospice-specific elements of care has been a large factor in inhibiting the utilization and accessibility of hospice services. Through 1981, the lack of uniform standards for hospice care, as well as the lack of conclusive evidence on cost savings, presented formidable obstacles to hospice coverage. However, 1982 and 1983 have been marked by significant expansion

TABLE 3-1
FRANK B. HALL CONSULTING CO.
HOSPICE SURVEY HIGHLIGHTS

	AETNA	BLUE CROSS/ BLUE SHIELD*	CONNECTICUT GENERAL	EQUITABLE
1. Hospice Coverage	Yes	71%	Yes	Yes
2. Separate Hospice Benefit Contract Rider **	Yes	Varies By Plan	Developing	Yes
a. Effective Date of Hospice Benefit	1982	Varies By Plan	--	1981
3. Premium Increase	No	2 Plans	N/A	No
4. Covered Services - a. Home Care Visits	Yes	Varies	Yes	Yes
b. Respite Care	No	By	Developing	Yes
c. Bereavement Counseling	No	Plan	Developing	Yes
5. Deductibles and Coinsurance Requirements	Same as Major Medical	Varies By Plan	Same as Major Medical	No
6. Limits	30 days Inpatient $3,000 Other Expenses Maximum	Varies By Plan	Developing	$5,000 Maximum

*   Figures are based upon the number of respondents to the internal Blue Cross/Blue Shield survey.
**   In addition to providing coverage under a defined benefit, many carriers reimburse hospice care as an expansion of existing benefits.
***   Reprinted with permission.
Information current 1983

in the area of hospice reimbursement. By 1982, carriers had begun reimbursing hospices even though standards and data still were lacking. Apparently, competitive pressure exists among carriers to evaluate and consider cost-effective alternatives to acute care for terminally ill patients.

Over the past three years, the Frank B. Hall Consulting Company has been tracing the development of private insurance reimbursement for hospice care. (Frank B. Hall Consulting Co., 1983; Berger-Friedman, 1983).

TABLE 3-1 (cont.)
FRANK B. HALL CONSULTING CO.
HOSPICE SURVEY HIGHLIGHTS

HARTFORD	HANCOCK	METROPOLITAN	MUTUAL OF OMAHA	NEW ENGLAND
Yes	Yes	Yes	Yes	Yes
Yes	Yes	Yes	Yes	Developing
1983	1983	1982	1982	--
No	Varies By Benefit Design	No	No	N/A
Yes Not specified Yes	Yes Flexible Flexible	Yes Yes Yes	Yes Developing Yes	Yes Developing Developing
No	Flexible	No	Same as Major Medical	To Be Developed
$100 Bereavement Counseling	Flexible	$7,500 Room & Board $3,000 Ancillary $500 Bereavement Counseling	None Specified	Developing

*   Figures are based upon the number of respondents to the internal Blue Cross/Blue Shield survey.
**   In addition to providing coverage under a defined benefit, many carriers reimburse hospice care as an expansion of existing benefits.
***   Reprinted with permission.
Information current 1983

TABLE 3-1 (cont.)
FRANK B. HALL CONSULTING CO.
HOSPICE SURVEY HIGHLIGHTS

	NEW YORK LIFE	PROVIDENT L & A	PRUDENTIAL	TRAVELERS
1. Hospice Coverage	Yes	71%	Yes	Yes
2. Separate Hospice Benefit Contract Rider **	Yes	Yes	Yes	Yes
a. Effective Date of Hospice Benefit	1983	1983	1982	1982
3. Premium Increase	No	No	No *Except* Medicare Eligibles	No
4. Covered Services -				
a. Home Care Visits	Yes	Yes	Yes	Yes
b. Respite Care	Yes	Not specified	Yes	Yes
c. Bereavement Counseling	Yes	Yes	Yes	Yes
5. Deductibles and Coinsurance Requirements	No *except* on plans with $500 or more deductible	50% of Covered Expenses	No	Same as Major Medical 50% for Bereavement Counseling
6. Limits	31 days Inpatient 100 Home Care Visits $50/visit for Bereavement Counseling	$5,000 Maximum	$3,000 (Maximum $150/day) Inpatient $2,000 Outpatient $200 Bereavement Counseling	Bereavement Counseling - 15 visits

*   Figures are based upon the number of respondents to the internal Blue Cross/Blue Shield survey.
**   In addition to providing coverage under a defined benefit, many carriers reimburse hospice care as an expansion of existing benefits.
***   Reprinted with permission.
Information current 1983

Table I reveals a summary of the Frank B. Hall Consulting Co.'s Research Paper--1983 Hospice Reimbursement Survey. It appears from Hall's successive surveys that there has been a growing trend toward a separately defined "hospice" benefit or contract rider which offers a comprehensive range of services. This introduces the element of coordination for management since most hospice services would be reimbursed under a single benefit. A freestanding hospice benefit will facilitate an insurance company's ability to identify utilization experience of the benefit.

Hospice planners and managers need to research any specific regulations within their state. Licensure provisions vary from state to state. Presently,* nineteen states have been reported to have enacted statutes which address hospices. They are as follows:

- California
- Colorado
- Connecticut
- Delaware
- Florida
- Georgia
- Hawaii
- Illinois
- Iowa
- Kentucky
- Maryland
- Massachusetts
- Michigan
- Nevada
- New York
- North Dakota
- Texas
- Virginia
- West Virginia

---

* As of Summer of 1984.

States have a viable option of creating hospice regulations through departments of health without passage of special hospice laws. Washington also has a varied type of state regulation. West Virginia has defined hospice in the context of a bill which sets up a state-wide continuum of care board. According to the legislative intent of this bill, the purpose of this board is to establish, encourage, and promote the availability and delivery of services within the state to the elderly, disabled, and the terminally ill and their families (Frank B. Hall Consulting Co., 1983). Blum and Robbins (1982) emphasize that the growing hospice field must address the need for licensure at state and national levels. Existing state laws and model bills and programs can help devise regulatory strategies for hospice. They give four primary reasons for hospice licensure:

- The need for the state to protect the public by guaranteeing that a given provider is offering services of acceptable quality

- The need to provide a legal basis of operation

- The need to evaluate reimbursement considerations based on the linkage between licensure and reimbursement

- The need to remove numerous ambiguities from hospice operations.

It is interesting to note that Connecticut, a jurisdiction viewed as a leader in the hospice field, has developed extensive hospice regulations on the basis of rather narrow legislation concerning insurance coverage for home care agencies. Maryland hospice legislation is noteworthy because they have developed a detailed set of regulations that requires all health insurance policies providing benefits on an expense-incurred basis to offer hospice care coverage as an optional benefit. The Florida statute passed in 1978 is the most detailed hospice licensure law in the country to control the organization and delivery of hospice services. The Florida law specifies the services a hospice must provide, staffing requirements, administrative structure, record-keeping and confidentiality procedures, and a yearly licensure requirement, as well as a special certificate-of-need provision, and admission by a licensed physician depend upon the express request and informed consent of patients and their families. Florida does not limit hospice care to terminally ill patients whose prognosis is less than one year. Hospice of Pa., Inc., a nonprofit private organization, also shares this view that hospice is appropriate for those suffering from life-threatening, incurable, lingering diseases. Ten states have certificate of need for hospice care.*

Many problems exist in defining the exact nature of the hospice concept in a manner that can be adequately reflected in regulations. States still need to

---

* Data current as of Spring 1984.

develop some type of regulatory strategy to protect both hospice programs and the public, and to enhance acceptability of hospices to paying parties. Again, by being creative, each area needs to develop its own hospice concept to meet local needs and to fit realistically into its own particular health care delivery system. According to Carol Bellamy, president of the council of the city of New York, the expansion of hospice is one of eight factors for cost containment noting that there are only fourteen *licensed* hospices in New York State (Bellamy, 1984).

Hospice persons involved in licensure give a list of licensure mistakes:

- state not involved in first draft

- exemption clauses

- grandfathering clause

In contrast, the following lists positive licensure points:

- use broad brush stroke to include all models

- use minimum standards

- does open up small party payors

- hire lobbyist (short term)

- look on drafting regulations also; don't start with licenses.

As a first step, Pennsylvania Hospice Network in December, 1984, adopted minimum standards for their state organization to use in recognizing hospice programs. Minimum standards are necessary to promote quality hospice care and should be adopted from JCAH (Joint Commission on Accreditation of Hospitals) Hospice Standards and NHO (National Hospice Organization) Standards to include patient and family as a unit of care, interdisciplinary team services, continuity of care, home care services, inpatient services, volunteer services, bereavement services, medical records, governing body, management and administration, and access to care.

A review of the literature reveals varied opinions about control systems such as operational protocols. However, the consensus agrees that flexibility is important, so that each hospice program can create its own structure, including details of organization, administration, services, and staffing.

Hospice of Pa., Inc., was among the first hospices in the country to receive certification under Medicare for the hospice benefit under the administration of this writer. The conditions of participation were reviewed under the section on hospice funding in Chapter 2. This first certification was possible because, as a community-based model, all the components required in order to qualify were already in place. The hospice must provide professional management responsibilities for all care rendered, even for care by outside providers. In terms of organization and administration, the already established linkages with management protocols among community providers is an excellent base for the Medicare certification application process. The process requires hospice directors to study the final regulations and respond accordingly. Strategies for professional management compliance will vary among models of care. As of July 20, 1984, 158 surveys for Medicare certification had been conducted. One hundred-one hospices had been certified in twenty-nine states with the largest number in Florida. Twelve hospices had withdrawn their applications and five had been denied. Forty programs are pending. As of that date, forty-one surveys had been scheduled (National Hospice Organization, 1984).* The new rules' financial and legal requirements will force hospices to carefully consider the risks and opportunities of the new Medicare hospice benefit (American Hospital Association, 1984). The regulations have apparently deterred the rural and smaller volunteer-based hospices from seeking certification. However, some larger hospices also decline to apply for reasons of economic feasibility. National Hospice Organization believes that only 25 percent of the nation's hospices can qualify for reimbursement at present (Sewell, 1984a).

Don Gaetz, former chairman of the National Hospice Organization (NHO) and the Rev. Hugh Westbrook have established a new for-profit hospice corporation that will seek Medicare reimbursement. The two hospice leaders have formed a $5 million corporation called Hospice Care, Inc., headquartered in Miami, which is being financed by bankers, entrepreneurs, and investment venture specialists. In a four-year plan, Gaetz states, the corporation projects that it will manage twelve to fifteen newly-created hospices across the country and will also offer a consulting service to help other hospices qualify for Medicare benefits. He also said that the company will set aside a large sum for indigent care, and that 47 percent of the ownership of the company will be allocated to its employees (Sewell, 1984b).

Gaetz and Westbrook led the fight two years ago to include hospice benefits in the Medicare program. Gaetz states that the new Medicare payment system daily rate of $46.25 is too low to cover costs at any but the largest hospices-- those that care for at least 100 people at a time. About 75 percent of hospices have fewer than twenty people enrolled at a time. Moreover, the system does not provide any special funds to cover the startup costs of a new hospice (Rich, 1984). NHO will be seeking higher rates from Congress, with a proposed increase from the current $46.25 to $53.17 for daily routine home care (Sewell, 1984a).** A single patient requiring long-term hospitalization or a patient needing expensive drugs, oxygen, and durable medical equipment at home would easily incur costs which would jeopardize a program's survival.

---

* At a recent seminar entitled "Financing Hospice," sponsored by Health Resources Publishing (March, 1985), Congressman Willis D. Gradison reported that only 165 hospices had been certified, with 50 more having applied and awaiting certification (out of 1300 hospices) (Sewell 1985).

** Rate increase effective October 1, 1984.

According to Edith Lohr, director of River Valley Hospice in Fargo, North Dakota--the first Medicare-certified hospice west of the Mississippi--the certification has been a good revenue-producing mechanism for their freestanding facility. Based on the experiences of a few hospices, programs can maximize this benefit and other supplemental insurance whenever possible in order to expand services and provide a more comprehensive program. In turn, it is saving the Medicare program money because of decreasing the number of inpatient hospital days. Hospitals and inpatient hospices must join forces in an effort to increase revenues and provide quality and more comprehensive services to the terminally ill patients and families.

Hospice is now being viewed by business coalitions, industry, health professionals, and hospital administrators as an alternative delivery system along with health maintenance organizations and preferred provider organizations. Business, labor, and provider leaders have recognized the importance of the containment of health care costs. It is increasingly clear that alternative health delivery systems do increase competition and introduce marketplace incentives to contain health care costs. The advantages of hospice must be explored on the basis of cost, quality, access to care, benefits, and delivery system characteristics. Consumers need hospice as an alternative to traditional structured health plans.

Other Sources. Hospice boards and administrators must continue to look beyond reimbursement mechanisms. Funding must be located for noncovered services and for the indigent who have no payment resources, as well as for start-up funds for program development. Traditional as well as new approaches may be used.

- Contracts for available federal, state, and local funds such as Title XX* for counseling and homemaker services

- Special demonstration projects with third-party payors such as Blue Cross

- Local, state, and national foundations (See foundation directories in any local library.)

- Private contributions such as banks or businesses

- Individual donations

- Memorial fund

- Application for grants from request for proposals from Federal Register and State Bulletins.

Staffing can also be enhanced through special programs. Organizations such as Area Agency for Aging and National Council for Aging provide funds for employment of individuals age fifty-five and over. This is a service of the

---

* Now Adult Service Block Grants.

Older Workers Employment Service. The workers may be hired in a hospice to do clerical work, maintenance, or to act as a driver or receptionist.

Each community will have access to a variety of funds, personnel, and other resources to supplement volunteer and staff services.

Establish Referral Sources

Unless hospice administrators establish appropriate linkages with community agencies and various facilities in the community to bring the hospice program closer to existing and future patients, referrals will be limited and other providers will come forth as competitors rather than supporters. A framework must be developed to assure these relationships.

One method is to identify a hospice registered nurse and medical social worker as hospice coordinators. Their major role would be to respond to calls for hospice services once the program is underway. Initially, however, the coordinators as a team would assist in establishing a procedure within each provider setting for facilitating referrals and completing the initial assessments-- medical, nursing (physical assessment), and psychosocial. Hospice coordinators must be skilled at public relations since their contacts and rapport with other professionals will often determine if hospice receives timely and appropriate referrals. Participation in patient care conferences and discharge planning meetings in hospitals helps educate the health care team members outside of hospice about hospice services and explains how the hospice as an organization can meet the needs of individuals and families. Educational programs for nursing and social work supervisors and their staff in the traditional settings is imperative to hospice success. These individuals are at the pivotal point where physicians are influenced and referral decisions are made.

More important, the extent to which hospice practices and philosophy of care become an established part of the health care system in a community rests with the physicians and the power of their referral capacities and their medical staff organizations.

Community agencies who host through educational programs are also good referral sources. Word-of-mouth is an important source for referrals, and is enhanced by the provision of good services. Referral sources for one month in one hospice are:

Physician--12%

Patient/family--13%

Hospital--75%

If referral sources are not secure, the hospice program may not survive.

Initiate Public Relations

A communication and education network established early in the planning stage provides a base for hospice acceptance. Traditional news media sources-- newspaper, radio, television--can tell the story very effectively. Interviews, stories about services, public service announcements, articles on hospice programs, and panel discussions are a few of many approaches. Human interest stories can demonstrate the *caring attitude* of hospice staff.

An agency newsletter with a creative format stimulates and informs the staff, board, committees, and public of services and activities of hospice.

NHO declares National Hospice Week the week following the NHO Annual Meeting in November each year. Each individual state can then plan a joint program through their state organization. Activities include a proclamation from the governor and area mayor, a series of newspaper articles, and a display in malls and downtown store fronts. The hospice public relations subcommittee should be expanded to include representatives from all media. An initial meeting with these representatives to educate them and tell the hospice story should be followed by quarterly meetings to discuss, develop a calendar of events, and implement an annual public relations program. Consider public relations needed for a year in advance and then decide relative usage of the different tools.

Hospices should become involved with spring festivals, career days, senior citizens days, ethnic festivities, educational forums and events, and other community activities throughout the year.

Hospice stickers, pins, bumper stickers, brochures, a traveling display--for example, a new building model--annual reports, information packets, and fact sheets should be circulated throughout the year. Any fundraising activities add to the public relations endeavors. Promotional tools also help acquire referrals; serve as a surrogate hospice spokesperson; clarify hospice services, philosophy, and policy; inform and educate health care professionals and the public; address competition; recruit staff and volunteers; help form acceptable attitudes and opinions among targets; and reflect the organization's managerial skills (Rubright and MacDonald, 1981).

Presentations to community groups--service clubs, PTAs, churches, women's clubs, professional organizations, and business groups--require a coordinator and a speakers bureau. Hospice staff must provide initial training sessions and ongoing information meetings for members of the speakers bureau. Slides, films, videotapes, audiotapes, and other similar tools are excellent audiovisual aids for a presentation. Educational workshops, seminars, special classes, and joint projects also need to be developed.

Involvement of the hospice administrator in community activities, as well as on state and federal hospice committees, helps keep the hospice informed on innovations elsewhere.

The hospice receptionist and office staff are responsible for giving the community a positive image of hospice in their daily telephone calls and visits from the public. Finally, each hospice staff member in his or her daily work with the health professionals and patients/families is the best public relations tool. One letter received from a patient's pastor states this very well:

> Let me express my appreciation for the high quality of the work done by Hospice. As Mrs. P.'s illness became progressively more severe and as the options available to her and her family became fewer and fewer, your Hospice nurses and counselors came as a breath of fresh air and hope. In their relationship with the P.'s, they gave service "above and beyond the call of duty." I was most particularly impressed with their care on the day Ann died. As one who has had some training and many occasions to be involved with the dying and their families, I appreciated the skill and knowledge of the death and dying process exhibited especially as they worked with the four young children. I had most contact with registered nurses but know from the family that the bereavement counselor also contributed much to the stability and peace of the family in a difficult time. As a pastor whose skills and abilities can only cover a limited area of the need faced by a family in a situation such as experienced by the P.'s. I can only say that I thank God for the love and grace shown by these members of your organization. I look forward to leaning upon your resources as occasion demands in the future.

Promoting the hospice and its programs can be targeted through three separate primary markets: the physician, the current and future patients and their families, and the community at large. Several people can be reached through the same promotional efforts while others are reached through spinoffs of these efforts. Use of the hospice care coordinators as liaison to the physicians' offices helps make the physician's clerical and nursing staff aware of the special services and programs within hospice. Patient/family support groups effectively highlight the hospice program as well.

In summary, marketing professionals generally agree that the main promotional channels in human services organizations are advertising, publicity, selling, and sales promotion. It is evident that consistent use of the publicity route is more prevalent among smaller organizations. Publicity, therefore, is the most enduring promotional channel, the least expensive, and easiest to use for hospices. The section which follows discusses marketing in relation to community support.

Nurture Community Support

The inclusion of a myriad of community people on the various hospice committees allows both input and a marketing nucleus. Hospice appointments to board committees must include health and other professionals including lawyers, realtors, engineers, bankers, accountants, and representatives from educational institutions, church groups, service clubs, auxiliaries, business, labor, industry, news media, and the consumer--a real cross-section of the community.

Marketing of hospice is a conceptual approach and a philosophy which permeates all levels of hospice activities from strategy to operations, affecting the organization of services as well as actual patient care. Based on Kotler (1980), marketing at the strategic level is a tool for survival, a means of integrating environmental trends and opportunities within the goals of hospice. On a tactical level, marketing is a process of social exchange. Its principles are applied in developing hospice services, the organizational model for delivery, and a program of action to promote hospice and motivate individuals to use its services. An expanded concept of marketing provided by Kotler is the analysis, planning, implementation, and control of carefully formulated programs designed to bring about voluntary exchanges of values with target markets for the purpose of achieving organizational objectives (Kotler, 1975). Marketing, with its explicit concern for resource allocation and public acceptance, can provide a planning and management tool for hospice managers (Cooper, 1979). According to Rubright and MacDonald (1981), when introducing marketing into the public relations operation one must be alert to the differences between public relations and marketing. Several points distinguish marketing from public relations, at least in health and human services.

Marketing is a planned strategy-oriented system of achieving objectives, which focuses on meeting the needs of patients through programs; public relations is public-oriented and is a tool to communicate messages dependent on the will, as well as mood, of the media persons (Rubright and MacDonald, 1981).

The 1984 Governor's Conference on Alternate Health Delivery Systems in Hershey, Pa. focused on Health Maintenance Organizations (HMOs), Preferred Provider Organizations (PPOs), and hospices as cost-effective alternatives. The emphasis, however, is on organization and administration and changes in practice management. Management must know about problems in target areas, demographic shifts, and other changes in the environment that could contribute to the evolution of hospice. Hospice administrators armed with comparative information on price, service, and quality must step forth and negotiate in the competitive market. More and more, hospice administrators will need to take an aggressive approach to inclusion of hospice in health benefit packages and HMOs.

In promoting hospice as a component of an HMO or PPO and as an extended benefit in existing health benefit programs, marketing strategies do include cost-effectiveness and quality services with added components such as a psychosocial approach and spiritual and bereavement counseling. Employees like to see added benefits in print; therefore, providing a brochure is imperative. Employee assistance programs also find the hospice service appealing, since it allows individuals to become productive again outside the home.

Community support letters demonstrate the value of hospice services to the community and emphasis should be placed on the model of care.

Sample letter from hospital administrator:

The philosophy of hospice care is to provide the patient, family, and community in general with an alternative to having quality comprehensive interdisciplinary team care for individuals diagnosed with a terminal disease. It is unlike any existing health care institution available to these terminal patients. A hospice program offers patient and families an opportunity for admission in order to stabilize patients medically; provide training to families and primary care providers in the unique aspects of caring for the terminally ill; and provide continuity of care allowing a discharge planning inpatient component to allow patients to return to their home environment whenever possible.

Sample letters from physicians:

The type of patient referred to the hospice program by me or in concurrence with others' choice, is one whose diagnosis no longer benefits from known treatment means and will show gradual deterioration and termination over whatever period remains.

The program is sound, the philosophy is in keeping with the highest ethical standards of the professionals involved, and the community requires its continued development to meet our human service needs. My intention is to continue utilizing all hospice services for my patients who will benefit.

As an oncologist, I utilize hospice services. The program has been of significant help for me in managing terminally ill patients with cancer and also sophisticated oncological problems. I feel there is a need for a skilled facility for hospice work. I will continue to utilize the hospice program as a referral source. The entire program in the country and especially in our area has been of great assistance to the management of patients with advanced cancer. I have contributed to the fundraising program last year.

Hospice has been providing excellent care to many of my patients at all hours of the day and night. This care is delivered with marvelous empathy and by professionals who are extremely qualified to render it. As a medical oncologist, I must say that this dimension is one that was sorely needed prior to the inception of hospice. We have so many patients who are suffering from terminal cancer in this region that clearly a comprehensive approach is one which must be energetically pursued.

I have referred many of my terminally ill patients to hospice for various reasons. The around-the-clock services provided to patients in need of home care is of the highest quality and delivered by a well-organized team of reliable nurses.

I am a busy family practitioner and can vouch for the need for continued hospice services for the countless cancer, cardiac, and other patients I have who are terminally and/or chronically ill and rely on hospice for help.

I am writing in support of this hospice organization as a local practicing physician. Our particular area is unfortunately subject to an unusually high proportion of cancer patients as a result of the unusually high number of elderly individuals living in this area. At present, we do have a number of home health care services competing with each other to aid these individuals. Nevertheless, it is my definite impression that the hospice organization has been the most effective in the outpatient support of terminally ill individuals particularly with malignancies. As you are aware, the hospice group is particularly organized to care for these unfortunate individuals and they have certainly lived up to their expectations in this area. I have heard numerous good reports from patients and families who have been referred to hospice for this type of care. At this point, however, we have a serious need for inpatient facilities for this type of patient. With restrictions in funding through Medicare, I am beginning to find myself frequently faced with terminal cancer patients who are unable to leave an inpatient environment because of the level of care required, and whose hospital expenses far exceed the amount apportioned by Medicare. It would seem to me that the hospice inpatient concept is the logical answer . . .

Sample letters from educational institutions:

With our own programs in physical therapy, nursing, human services and psychology here at the University, we would not only be in a position but would welcome the opportunity to work cooperatively with hospice. We believe that the people of this region genuinely need this kind of professional assistance.

We feel that our students and the patients and families with whom they will become involved as caregivers will be mutually enriched by their participation in an expanded hospice program that includes an inpatient facility as well as home care.

We feel grateful that it is possible for our students to participate in the "total needs" approach to caregiving that the hospice members involved with the home care phase of the hospice program as interns, volunteers, or board members. We want our students to have an opportunity to be of service to the elderly, persons with multiple chronic illnesses, and the terminally ill.

I see the need among our human services majors for a practicum of the type which hospice facility will provide. The hospice philosophy, emphasizing as it does the value of life and the dignity of the person even in stages of physical breakdown of long-term and terminal nature, is a valuable perspective for future providers of a wide variety of human services. I see a great potential in the availability of hospice for training and research, as well as for direct care.

While hospice care is still a rarity in this country, I believe we will begin to see the cost-effectiveness of the combination of hospital, home care, and hospice care for certain types of patients. After there are examples existing on which studies can be done, I am certain that we will come to accept hospice care as a viable health care alternative.

Our committee of the Hospice Foundation is exerting much energy on fundraising efforts, and once the hospice program expands, we look forward to obtaining grants from major sources.

This project has my wholehearted support both for the elderly ill of our area, and for the educational potential it has for college students and other health care providers.

Sample letters from community groups:

After much discussion and deliberation, the members of our auxiliary decided to direct our financial support toward Hospice and their efforts. The projects already undertaken and those in the planning state meet the needs of both the youth and elderly of our community, and the new inpatient beds will widen the horizon of the Hospice program.

Chronically ill residents are provided with personal care, transportation to services necessary for their care, and companionship when family members are unavailable. The bereavement counseling has eased the pains of death to many local families.

It is our hope as an auxiliary to contribute financially and through volunteers become an important part of the Hospice program.

As President of a building and construction trades council, I represent some five thousand building and construction tradesmen in a nine county area.

Our members and their families have taken an active role in our community and are particularly interested in adequate health care.

It is with this in mind that we have been involved with the hospice program. The various trade unions have pledged money toward the development of a hospice facility, and through our apprenticeship and training programs, we have helped to renovate the office facilities for hospice home care.

Many of our members' families have used the hospice concept and have informed me of the warmth and care which is administered through the program at a very difficult time in their lives.

On behalf of all of the tradesmen and their families, I want to inform you that we are totally supportive of the hospice program and we see a definite need for such a program in our community.

Sample letters from churches:

There is no doubt in my mind that hospice care is clearly needed in our area. It will fill a gap in medical and emotional care that is not currently being met by any other type of skilled nursing care unit. I know of no member of the clergy in this area who has in any way been displeased with the quality of care hospice has given. In my own parish I once counted more than 40 persons who had cancer, several of whom have benefitted from hospice care and concern.

Certainly the ministries of Hospice has been of great benefit to the dying and to their families. In my experience I have found that short term confinement is frequently necessary when one or more of the other members need care and nursing homes or hospitals are not available. In addition, I am convinced that there would be better nursing home or hospital utilization if such short-term care were available to demonstrate the efficacy of more adequate care; and on the other hand to provide a training period for family members so they might do a better job when the sick person comes home.

Sample letters from politicians:

As you know, hospice deals directly with cancer victims, the elderly, and their families in providing sensitive and continued care. It is a very unique concept and there is a definite need for a program such as this. Hospice has been well-received and is supported by area hospitals, physicians, and the community in general.

We county commissioners have supplied a rent-free office to hospice in our Court House Annex since 1979 and we have had first hand observances of the growth and needs of the organization.

City Council is pleased and honored to join the increasing number of people who are dedicating themselves to hospice. May it be our good fortune to make some meaningful contribution to the success of the hospice program.

Sample letters from individuals:

I have been motivated to offer financial support by seeing the work they do first hand. They truly exemplify the adage: "Find a need and fill it."

The whole concept of hospice is magnificent. It provides dignity to dying and keeps people whole. But beyond this much needed philosophy and actual program, hospice appears to have broad-based support from all who have encountered its wonderful work.

Marketing can be used to bring the hospice and its services to the attention of the public. The foundation of all marketing theory is exchange. Simply put, it means that the hospice manager comes together in the marketplace with other caregiving resources in the community to coordinate services. Rubright and MacDonald (1981) use an example of this exchange.

A nursing home decides to open a hospice section for the terminally ill; along the way, it must inform patients and their families of the new offering.

What exchange is involved between the hospice and the patient/family unit? (a) The nursing home hospice offers space in an existing medical facility, extraordinary concern for the problems of the patient and the family, rigid control of pain and symptoms, a contemporary approach to death and dying, 24-hour support service, and physical and emotional comfort. (b) The patient/family unit receives the benefits of and pays for the service, endorses the hospice concept, possibly makes contributions to the institution, offers encouragement to the staff. Family members may even volunteer their time. With such an exchange (the nursing home gives a little more than the user) it is small wonder that the hospice movement is advancing so steadily in the United States.

Each hospice manager must martial all the forces in their individual community and, on the basis of responses, seek to meet the health care needs of the community through an appropriate model for hospice care.

Population, news media, and management changes are evidence that the first law of ecology--everything is connected to everything else--may also apply to a hospice program. With hospice in constant interaction with the environments, it is highly important to reckon with the appropriate forces in the community. Marketing is community-oriented; the organization is integral, working part of a changing, dynamic environment. Advocacy and participation are important to the success of hospice (Rubright and MacDonald, 1981).

Evaluate and Research

Evaluation of hospice program components must be carried out on an annual basis or more often if necessary. Program evaluation becomes a responsibility of staff, committee, and board members. Through an annual report and self-evaluation process the coordinator/supervisor of each service writes an annual summary which narrates the activities of the year and reflects on any changes and/or developments for the coming year. Hospice administration then analyzes this report with middle-management and with the professional advisory committee who then makes recommendations to the board. Program evaluation becomes a part of the total quality assurance program which will be discussed further in Chapter 4. Day-to-day working integration of administration and evaluation provides a seamless dynamic interaction necessary for hospice programming (White, 1981).

One community-based model carries out an evaluation of its program by having each patient complete a form. The survey is designed for families who have participated in the program and is used to promote quality care. The survey includes the following:

    A. **ADMISSIONS**
        1. Prompt response to initial inquiry
        2. First explanation of the program
        3. Courtesy of counselor and/or nurse responding to inquiry

B. SERVICE
1. Response to your loved one's medical needs
2. Response to your loved one's nursing needs
3. Response to your family's emotional needs
4. In your opinion--response to the emotional needs of your loved one
5. Response to your family's spiritual needs
6. In your opinion--response to the spiritual needs of your loved one
7. Dependability of after-hour's service
8. Promptness of response in emergencies

C. SUPPORTIVE SERVICES
1. Assistance in obtaining special equipment
2. Assistance in meeting the need for special services such as:
   Transportation
   Family relief/respite care
   Errands
3. Response to your needs at time of your loved one's death
4. Continued contact during bereavement

One hospice has a program evaluation format to meet function requirements which involves board and committee review of administration, services, staffing, and finance. Written policies and statistics are reviewed annually focusing on the four areas.

JCAH Accreditation provides both a self-evaluation mechanism and a tool for research. The hospice medicare regulation requires that all participating hospice organizations file cost reports with HCFA. The accumulation of such cost statistics will provide the widest body of information yet assembled on hospice characteristics, utilization, and costs. This data base will be helpful in further research. Because of mandated data collection and analysis, the assumptions, misconceptions, myths, and true values of hospices will be able to be objectively assessed (Amenta, 1984).

Hospice care is an excellent setting for research projects because it blends existing disciplines to achieve one goal so that care can be administered holistically. There are limited studies on the effects of counseling the death and dying and their families, the outcomes of a bereavement program, the approaches to care of the chronically ill and elderly, the use of volunteers in health care, the family and patient as a "single unit of care," and the numerous other aspects of care which hospice brings, for the first time, to the health care system. Since hospice may be an agent for change in the American health care delivery system, hospice managers must be alert to the extremely important role of hospice in future research. Research into satisfaction indexes of patients, families, and professionals is also vital to hospice programs. The outcomes of hospice care in relation to the ability of the family to cope in the future must be studied. Initial research questions might be: What impact does hospice care have on decreasing family problems and lowering the incidence of disease conditions among family members? Does hospice care decrease teenage suicide? Does hospice care reduce the incidence of alcoholism and drug abuse in family members after the patient died? Has hospice care increased the lifetime of a surviving spouse? Has hospice care decreased the mortality rate within the two years after the patient's death of an *elderly* surviving spouse?

Hospice administrators must continually assess the need for further research and development of high quality and cost-effective programs. Involvement of the educational facilities (as indicated in sample letters in the previous section on community support) is certainly a tremendous advantage for the research component of hospice care in a university setting.

A hospice administrator who is attentive to these "ten commandments" may tell his or her staff that hard work will lead to success. Indeed, this theory of reward being commensurate with effort has been an enduring belief in our society.

Quality hospice services are delivered efficiently in an everchanging environment of government regulations, consumer activism, and budget limitations through education, research, observation and, most important, practice. The hospice management must bring knowledge, committment and quality to the hospice organization. The hospice manager must be competent in management techniques and he or she must comprehend both social and technical systems. The manager must also possess interpersonal skills, not the least of which is the ability to defer his or her own immediate desires and gratifications in order to cultivate the talents of others (Levey and Loomba, 1973).

The supervisor, or coordinator in many hospice programs are often clinicians who face a role change from direct service work to middle-management. Often the nurse or social worker was a traditional caregiver who assisted in starting the hospice program because of a belief in hospice philosophy. Frequently this person must monitor the effectiveness of hospice services and supervise the technical work of professional and nonprofessional subordinates. The qualities of communication, good judgement, maturity, initiative, dedication, committment and imagination that a nurse or social worker must possess are advantages in the movement into middle-management. In the new role, the supervisor must develop an understanding of formal organizational theory and the ways in which individuals and organizations interact in work and political settings. On becoming a manager, hospice professional caregivers should seek out educational opportunities to begin to learn more about the art and technology of management. As Dressler (1978) noted, if caregivers are unwilling to manage, then hospice programs of the future may be led by nonclinician bureaucratic administrators who may be more accountable to monolithic institutions than to the hospice health care professionals or to the hospice patients and families they serve. Hospice professionals are as much a constituency of the manager as are consumers. Chapter 4 on discusses this important aspect of hospice management.

Since the environment is changing rapidly, hospice programs will be forced to change their degree of complexity. A hospice manager needs to know the forces and factors at work and the need for effective strategies to deal with the broad range of management responsibilities. Application of the growing number of techniques and principles requires astute analysis for hospice practice.

REFERENCES

Amenta, Madalon. (1984). Reimbursement, accreditation and the movement's future: Hospice has initiated reform, but will it be lasting. *The American Journal of Hospice Care* 1(1):10-14.

American Hospital Association. (1984). Washington Report. Hospice programs move slowly to seek Medicare Certification. *Outreach* 5(2):4.

Argyris, Chris. (1957). *Personality and Organization.* New York: Harper and Bros.

_____. (1964). *Integrating the Individual and the Organization.* New York: John Wiley and Sons.

Bellamy, Carol. (1984). Paper presented at the Columbia University Seminar on Health Care: At What Cost? New York City, April 27.

Berger-Friedman, Patricia J. (1983) Paying for Hospice Care. *Hospitals* 57(16):106-108.

Blum, John D., and Dennis A. Robbins. (1982). Regulation. *Hospitals* 56(23): 91-94, 96.

Bunn, Elizabeth G. (1984). Volunteers as the backbone. *The American Journal of Hospice Care* 1(1):34-36.

Carr, Charles A., and Donna M. Carr. (1983). *Hospice Care Priniciples and Practice.* New York: Springer Publishing Company.

Cooper, Philip D. (1979). *Health Care Marketing Issues and Trends.* Rockville, MD: Aspen Systems Corporation.

Department of Health and Human Services, Health Care Financing Administration. 1982. Medicare Program; Comprehensive Outpatient

Rehabilitation Facility Services; Final Rule. *Federal Register.* December 15.

_____. (1983). Conditions of Participation for Hospice Benefits under Medicare. *Federal Register.* December 16.

Donovan, Judy A. (1984). Team Nurse and Social Worker--Avoiding Role Conflict. *The American Journal of Hospice Care* 1(1):21-23.

Dooley, Jeanne. (1982). The Corruption of Hospice. *Public Welfare.* (Spring): 35-41.

Dressler, D. M. (1978). Becoming an Administrator: The Vicissitudes of Middle Management in Mental Health Organizations. *American Journal of Psychiatry* 135(3):357-360.

Drucker, P. F. (1974). *Management: Tasks, Responsibilities and Practices.* New York: Harper and Row.

Frank B. Hall Consulting Company. (1983). *Hospice Reimbursement Survey.* Hawthorne, NY.

Freud, Sigmund. (1907/1959). *Mourning and Melancholia Collected Papers.* Vol. 4. New York: Basic Books.

Goldsmith, Seth B. (1981). *Health Care Management: A Contemporary Perspective.* Rockville, MD: Aspen Systems Corporation.

Graham, Nancy O., ed. (1982). *Quality Assurance in Hospitals.* Rockville, MD: Aspen Systems Corporation.

Herzberg, Frederick, Bernard Mausner, and Barbara Block Snyderman. (1959). *The Motivation to Work.* New York: John Wiley and Sons.

Kotler, Phillip. (1975). *Marketing for Nonprofit Organizations.* Englewood Cliffs, NJ: Prentice-Hall.

_____. (1980). *Marketing Management: Analysis, Planning, and Control.* Englewood Cliffs, NJ: Prentice-Hall.

Levey, Samuel, and Paul N. Loomba. (1973). *Health Administration.* Philadelphia: J.B. Lippincott Company.

Liebler, Joan Gratto, Ruth Ellen Levine, and Hyman Leo Dervitz. (1984). *Management Principles for Health Professionals.* Rockville, MD: Aspen Systems Corporation.

Maslow, Abraham. (1954). *Motivation and Personality.* New York: Harper and Row.

McCann, Barbara A. (1983). Hospice Care: A Challenge and an Opportunity for Discharge Planners. *American Hospital Association Discharge Planning Update* (Fall):8.

McCool, Barbara, and Montague Brown. (1977). *The Management Response: Conceptual, Technical and Human Skills of Health Administration.* Philadelphia: W.B. Saunders Company.

McGregor, Douglas. (1960). *The Human Side of Enterprise.* New York: McGraw-Hill.

McNulty, Elizabeth Gilman, and Robert A. Holderby. (1983). *Hospice: A Caring Challenge.* Springfield, IL: Charles C. Thomas.

Menapace, Nancy. (1982). *Proposal for Bereavement Program.* Hospice of Pennsylvania, Inc. Typescript.

National Hospice Organization. (1982). *Standards of a Hospice Program of Care.* Arlington, VA.

_____. (1984). *State Hospice Connection.* Arlington, VA.

Ouchi, William (1981). *Theory Z: How American Business Can Meet The Japanese Challenge.* Reading, MA: Addison-Wesley.

Pryga, Ellen A., and Henry J. Bachofer. (1983). *Hospice Care Under Medicare. A Working Paper.* Chicago: American Hospital Association, Office of Public Policy Analysis.

Rich, Spencer (1984). 2 Hospice Pioneers Starting a Business. *The Federal Report, The Washington Post,* February 22nd.

Rodek, Christine F., and Susan Jacob. (1983). Perspectives on Hospice. *Cancer Nursing* 6(3):183.

Rubright, Robert, and Dan McDonald. (1981). *Marketing Health and Human Services.* Rockville, MD: Aspen Systems Corporation.

Rush, Harold M. (1969). *Behavioral Science Concepts and Management Application.* New York: The Conference Board, Inc.

Sewell, Marshall, Jr. (1984a). Hospice Medicare Applications Continue to Lag. *Hospice Letter* 6(12).

_____. (1984b). Leader Forms For Profit Hospice Company. *Hospice Letter* 5(12).

Ufema, Joy. (1984). Personal Concerns of Hospice Movement. *The American Journal of Hospice Care* 1(1):5.

U. S. General Accounting Office. (1979). *Hospice Care--A Growing Concept in the United States.* HRD 79-50, March 6.

Wald, Florence S., Zelda Foster, and Henry J. Wald. (1980). The Hospice Movement As a Health Care Reform. *Nursing Outlook* 28(3):173-178.

White, Stephen L. (1981). *Managing Health and Human Service Programs: A Guide for Managers.* New York: The Free Press.

Zangwill, Willard I. (1976). *Success with People--The Theory Z Approach to Mutual Achievement.* Homewood, IL: Dow-Jones-Irwin.

Chapter 4

Quality of Hospice Care

Hospice programs bring to the health care delivery system a degree of excellence which has not always been met in traditional settings. Quality is defined as the basic nature which makes something what it is. In the 1970s, public accountability shaped decision-making in health care; the question of reimbursement was one of the major issues under discussion.

Traditional home care policy has been highly regulated in regard to structure and process but not with regard to quality and outcome. Publicly funded programs have had to focus on access and cost with limited concern for measurement of health status to determine the value of services. Quality is not linked with reimbursement in the Medicare structure and is not promoted by its payment policies (Mundinger, 1983). Since home care is a major component of hospice and many hospice programs have become certified home care programs, concerted effort must be made to assure that hospice characteristics are well implemented within each program and quality of care addressed from all perspectives, especially outcomes.

ELEMENTS OF QUALITY CARE

Initially, the hospice administrator must address the points discussed in Chapter 2--The "Ten Commandments." The hospice that is put into operation must provide the best possible array of needed services for each individual patient and family. Performance evaluation of individuals, departments, and management must be both program-focused and problem-focused.

High-quality hospice care depends heavily on attracting a high-quality staff. The traditional system of health care has failed to stimulate its most dedicated workers. "Overregulation" of the health care system has squelched improvisation. Therefore, many dissatisfied health professionals in conventional health care delivery have been drawn to the hospice program, where they are encouraged to combine their compassion and sensitivity with their basic technical skills to provide exceptional services (Miller, 1984).

In forecasting the use of hospice services, quality of care is easily one of the most important success criteria, although it is one of the most difficult to measure. Quality care can be addressed objectively by examination of resources used in patient care, the activities of patient care, or its outcomes. Quality can be measured subjectively by asking patients and professionals how they perceive the provider's quality of care.

Since the objective of hospice care is to enhance quality of life by attending to physical, spiritual, and psychological needs, examination of quality of hospice care requires an understanding of how hospice care works. Interdisciplinary hospice care works toward ensuring patient comfort; this requires a highly skilled, compassionate, and technically proficient team, which includes professional staff, family, close friends, and volunteers.

Elements of quality hospice care include the following:

- Professional management responsibility for *all* care.

- Primary staff assignments for continuity of care.

- Participation of patient/family in decision making.

- Provision for family members to stay with inpatients around the clock with no age or time restrictions on visiting hours.

- Use of home care when adequate.

- Imaginative care, unhurried, with attention to detail.

- Attention to practical, mundane concerns that matter--wet bed sheets, insomnia, bed positioning, feelings of isolation, skin care, and prevention of decubiti.

- Attention to dietary needs.

- Ability to perform tasks for patients such as feeding a patient with patience and devotion, not with a mind on other matters.

- Emphasis on symptom control and physical needs--control of nausea and vomiting, bowel and bladder function, and respiratory distress; alleviation of treatment side effects, such as pruritis, stomatitis, edema, elevated temperature, and altered mental state.

- Effective pain control which necessitates identification of etiology, prevention of pain before it appears, and administration of medication as simply as possible to allow the patient to self-administer drugs, maintain alertness, and live as normally as possible.

- A plan of care developed by the interdisciplinary team with ongoing assessment.

- Early collaboration among team members during development of the plan of care to clarify roles and a

unified approach since role blurring occurs within the
hospice care team.

- A staff that works well together--group consensus, same
approach, "concerted effort and thinking."

- A nurturing and secure environment with a daily
supportive system for families with familiar staff persons.

- A spiritual/humanistic approach which is, in many ways, a
medical self-help movement.

- Use of empathy in addition to support to understand
individual patients; an avoidance of stereotyping.

- Therapeutic communication among staff.

- Attention to the psychosocial evaluation as a guide for
intervention to bring the uniqueness of each individual
into focus.

- Careful coordination by the interdisciplinary team of
planning and interventions of *all* persons who have contact
with the terminally ill patient and his or her family.

- Volunteer services as a component of the interdisciplinary
team.

- Available individual and family counseling.

- An information/support/program for patients/families.

- An exceptional comprehensive orientation, in-service
training, and continuing education program for all staff
and volunteers.

- Continuing care team follow-up after the patient's death--
bereavement program.

As stated by Salloday (1984), one of the hallmarks of hospice care is its
conscious and consistent reliance on "people technology" in preference to
mechanical technology to provide quality patient care.

A hospice certainly offers distinct opportunities for physicians to practice
high quality medicine. However, equally important to quality care are the
physician's personal qualities, his or her academic training, the physician's work
within a competitive climate and the organizational environment. Physicians
who are better educated about the hospice concept of care are more likely to
enhance their medical management. Continuity of care from the hospice team
who follow the patient throughout the course of the disease allows staff members
the opportunity to build supportive relationships with patient and family
members. This enhances the security of a caring environment.

In order to establish the best organizational environment, hospice staff
support must be provided as needed in stressful situations. This support should
be supplemented by educational programs for staff training. The organizational

structure itself affects the quality of care provided by the varied hospice models, as evidenced by the research and experiences of the author.

THE IMPACT OF THE ORGANIZATION ON THE QUALITY OF CARE

Determination of impact is a very sophisticated process requiring careful research and continuing evaluation. It is important to build sound research and evaluation procedures into the structure of any new hospice program. Clearly defined goals and measurable objectives must be formulated as the first essential step in demonstrating the legitimacy, the effectiveness, and the value of any hospice program. Responsible evaluation will then seek to determine the extent to which these goals are being accomplished and what program changes or improvements are necessary. It is necessary to examine structure, which includes point of view, resources available, population to be served; process, which includes describing and analyzing procedures and services; and outcome, which seeks a testable design for evaluating the goal to be accomplished. Teamwork in administration at the top level is as essential as teamwork among the persons actually working with the patients if the objectives are to be accomplished.

Hospice practice should utilize natural systems as sources of help and change and should protect and nurture sources of support and opportunities for growth and self-realization that exist in a patient's human environment; hence the importance of home care in hospice.

Early in the development of any hospice program limitations on the number of patients is essential. Initially, only one patient/family should be accepted at a time until the hospice care team and administration are certain that all needed services are provided or coordinated on a comprehensive basis to meet the individual's needs. This is referred to as a minimum level of utilization. In contrast, utilization levels that overtax the capacity of space, equipment, and personnel cause reductions in quality. Forecasts of utilization help managers make decisions about whether appropriate quality can be maintained and what resources are necessary to do so.

The description and discussion of each hospice model in Part II focuses on what effect the organizational structure and administration of each model has on quality of care. The author's research and experiences reflect that the community-based model of hospice care with central administration and coordination is most effective as a private nonprofit agency in providing quality hospice care based on the hospice characteristics and elements of care discussed earlier.

Achieving improvement and quality of care through organizational change in an inpatient setting requires that hospice personnel learn new ideas and concepts, new attitudes and skills, and new patterns of behavior. This process of planned change is very difficult: present habits or practices must be unlearned and new beliefs, values, attitudes, and behavior patterns must be developed. Quality assurance programs may be viewed as managerial activities designed to enhance and facilitate the change process in health care institutions. New hospice programs within the inpatient setting require an ongoing evaluation and monitoring system in order to assure quality care.

Traditional home care programs are required to have a program evaluation available for use; therefore, the home care agency that has expanded into a hospice is already prepared in this area. However, traditional home care agencies such as visiting nurse associations have limited team resources and a lack of *formal* ties within the community limiting a hospice program within that structure to establish quality.

All hospice programs must be committed to developing and utilizing methods to measure and assure quality of patient/family care including evaluation of services, regular chart audits, and organizational review.

The Quality Assurance Program

The traditional definition of quality in health care includes both the technical, scientific aspect and the "art" of the care. The art of care refers to the manner in which members of the hospice care team conduct themselves in relation to their patient families. Quality is the optimal achievable result for each patient/family in a cost-effective way; it takes into account perspective, values, and purpose. Quality is dynamic; it changes as knowledge, values, and resources change.

The quality assurance program of a hospice exists to assess and encourage the best quality care for all patients and their families. Quality assurance is a dual process. It is the examination of the appropriateness and quality of clinical services as well as a process of education. It becomes an ongoing developmental and training tool to improve clinical skills and establish the levels of performance expected from all clinicians. The program strives to ensure that services provided meet accepted professional standards and that staff and services are utilized appropriately and effectively.

The quality assurance program involves the following components:

- Utilization Control

- Peer Review

- Clinical Record Review

- Patient Care Audit

- Program Evaluation

No one component is synonymous with quality assurance but rather each is an element of a well-founded quality assurance program. These components provide the structure by which quality assessment can be operationalized. Quality assessment and quality assurance are mutually interdependent aspects of the two-fold process of a quality assurance program. Quality assurance cannot be implemented as an operational reality without a refined process of assessing quality of care.

If there is only quality assessment, the predictable staff reactions would be resistance, confusion, and feelings of being threatened. Quality assessment uncomplemented by positive educational components is not quality assurance. The components of the quality assurance program provide the structure by which quality assessment can be operationalized, but these mechanisms do not guarantee the delivery of health care. It is only through the second dimension of these components, that is, the development, training, and mastering of clinical skills that quality care can be provided and maintained.

It becomes the responsibility of health care professionals to go beyond mere assessment, and encourage professional growth and development which, in turn, will be transferred into higher quality care for the consumer.

Quality assurance is not intended to objectify clinical judgment, promote stereotyped or standardized treatments for diverse problems, improve records, or vindicate status quo. Nor does quality assurance intend to merely serve as another form of bureaucratic compliance. Sound clinical judgment has parameters; treatment plans and programs have data bases; records have been formalized and these are necessary and operational parameters to any quality assurance program.

Quality assurance approaches are often mixed up with program evaluation, interpersonal staff relationships, reviews of the completeness of records, data base development, and formulation of written policies and procedures. Activities which are already mandated by accreditation, licensure, or reimbursement agencies have been inappropriately referred to as "quality assurance" even though they do not contain effective mechanisms for implementing change in patient care, service utilization, or staff resource maximization.

It seems appropriate for hospice administrators to set standards for care of the dying person then examine the care given in a manner similar to our traditional method of monitoring care to the sick, such as utilization review and patient care audits (Carr and Carr, 1983).

Utilization control becomes an area of focus in hospice care. Utilization review has been an important aspect of a quality assurance program in health care for some time now. Basically, utilization control is a concurrent review program that seeks to assure that the patient is receiving the appropriate level of care and for a reasonable length of time. Utilization control also combines efficiency and appropriate use of health care resources. Initially, the hospice admission team must ask the question--Is the hospice care appropriate for this patient? If appropriate, then the interdisciplinary team must provide an ongoing review to determine appropriateness of continued hospice care. Members of the interdisciplinary team serve as a utilization review committee. Utilization of hospice services is specific in the federal regulations for reimbursement. The hospice benefit under Medicare states that 80% of the patient days must be provided in the home setting and 20% in the inpatient setting. Utilization review is primarily concerned with the cost of care. The hospice team has the ongoing responsibility of determining which health resources are effective and adequate for hospice patients.

Peer review in hospice care becomes a voluntary review among peers. A detailed review of the plan of care on an informal daily basis and formally on a weekly basis among interdisciplinary team members is an approach for monitoring the quality of care. Peer review by colleagues does not fully meet the more rigorous requirements of a valid and reliable judgment on the quality of care. For that it is necessary to specify in detail the appropriate strategies of care as judged by their benefits, risks, and costs (Graham, 1982). The interdisciplinary team approach in hospice care strengthens the peer review process. Education of staff in practicing the team concept is a step toward ongoing peer review.

Self-evaluation as part of a performance evaluation process allows hospice caregivers to objectify the evaluation of their care to patients and opens the door for constructive comments and suggestions from peers. Peer review can also be sought by those outside of the hospice team. Often hospice home care staff will seek feedback from hospital caregivers and, in one instance, we have observed hospice staff approaching nurses in the physician's office to solicit comments about their hospice care. This type of peer review can be initiated only in a nonthreatening hospice environment.

Hospice managers rely on the interdisciplinary group for the development of a comprehensive plan of care, provision of the care, and continuous evaluation and revision of the plan of care. This inherently involves continuous peer review.

Clinical record review includes both utilization control and peer review. Upon admission and every thirty days thereafter, a member of the clinical record review team composed of RN supervisors must review each record focusing on specific criteria; that is, completion of an adequate assessment, completion of an appropriate care plan, implementation of care plan, determination of whether goals were met, and documentation of planning including discharge if appropriate. This process determines adequacy of the plan of treatment and appropriateness of continuation of care.

The clinical record review team specifically reviews the following areas and makes recommendations accordingly:

1. Patients are accepted for services on the basis of a reasonable expectation that the patient's medical, nursing, and social needs can be met adequately by hospice in the patient's place of residence.

2. Patient/family care follows a written plan of treatment established and periodically reviewed by a physician, and care continues under the general supervision of a physician.

3. The plan of treatment developed in consultation with the hospice care team covers all pertinent diagnoses, including:

- mental status

- types of services and equipment required

- frequency of visits

- prognosis

- rehabilitation potential

- functional limitations

- activities permitted

- nutritional requirements

- medications and treatments*

- any safety measures to protect against injury

- instructions for timely referrals; i.e., continuing care team (bereavement)

- laboratory procedures

- specialized procedures (Cormed pump, hyper-alimentation), any contraindications or precautions to be observed

- medical assessment, nursing assessment, and psychosocial evaluation

- orders for therapy services include the specific procedures and modalities to be used and the amount, frequency, and duration

- volunteer services

4. The hospice interdisciplinary care team who participates in developing the plan of treatment meets at least weekly to review the plan of care and recommends any charges as needed.

5. The hospice RN checks all medications a patient may be taking to identify possible ineffective drug therapy or adverse reactions, significant side effects, drug allergies, and contraindicated medication, and reports any problems to the physician.

6. A skilled summary is written monthly when care team visits exceed three per week or are made less than twice a month.

---

* Medication list must include side effects and skilled nursing observations/monitoring required with intervention when necessary.

Clinical record review is an ongoing process. A summary of the review and recommendations are recorded as a component of the medical record. The clinical record review team meets *once* every two weeks to analyze results and plan corrective action. Correction action involves a staff educational process and record form revisions when appropriate.

Patient care audit is supervised by the audit committee. This subcommittee of the professional advisory committee meets quarterly to review clinical records to assure that established policies are followed in providing services. The audit committee consists of health care professionals who represent each discipline on the hospice care team as follows: From the community: physician; registered nurse; medical social worker; physical therapist; speech therapist; nutritionist; psychiatrist; clergy; and pharmacist. From staff: RN supervisor; MSW supervisor; staff RN; staff social worker; and others as needed based on current audit, e.g., if cancer is diagnosed, an oncologist would be consulted.

The focus of each audit is determined by priorities: percentage of patients according to diagnosis, percentage of patients according to age, metastatic disease, symptoms (pain control and spinal decompression), complications (hypercalcemia), and others as needed based on findings of clinical record review team. Oncology nursing guidelines from the policy and procedure manual are integrated into this process.

Audits are conducted under the supervision of an RN supervisor specifically trained in quality assurance. The purpose is to measure the degree of excellence of the program against established criteria or standards.

Program Evaluation consists of assessment of outcomes of care to hospice patients through a formalized system of assessment review--while services are being provided and upon death or discharge for other reasons--evaluates results of service in terms of health status and patient satisfaction.

Besides the individual third-party payor requirements for providers of hospice care, two main types of activities address the question of standards governing the delivery of hospice care: state licensure and voluntary standards.

Two organizations have been actively involved in the development of standards for hospice care: National Hospice Organization and Joint Commission on Accreditation of Hospitals.

ACCREDITATION AND HOSPICE

For accreditation, the Joint Commission on Accreditation of Hospitals has included utilization review and quality assurance as standards in their *Hospice Standards Manual*. The quality assurance standard states that the hospice program strives to assure the provision of high quality patient/family care through the monitoring and evaluation of the quality and appropriateness of hospice program services (Joint Commission on Accreditation of Hospitals,

1983). Management and administrative staff are responsible for assuring the implementation and maintenance of a planned and systematic process and for resolving identified problems through a written plan. Any findings of the quality assurance program are a basis for action in the areas of patient/family services, administration or supervision, and in-service or continuing education. In addition, in some instances the medical record forms may need revisions or additions for ease of documentation.

The standard for utilization review states that the allocation of hospice resources is monitored and identified problems in the utilization of hospice resources are resolved. This requires ongoing monitoring of the utilization of home care, inpatient, and interdisciplinary team services.

Hospice Care Accreditation Program

Accreditation by the Joint Commission on Accreditation of Hospitals (JCAH) is recognized as a quality standard by most federal and state health regulatory agencies. JCAH accreditation symbolizes quality to the public and to the health care field. For hospice directors, accreditation provides a management tool. JCAH accreditation is based on practice standards rather than organizational standards because no one organizational model has been proven best as to cost and quality.

In 1981, JCAH was awarded a grant from the Kellogg Foundation to assess the state of the art of hospice care in America and to determine the need for voluntary hospice accreditation. Data resulting from several national surveys showed an overwhelming interest in hospice care accreditation. After extensive field review involving the participation of over 400 hospice programs, JCAH published the *Hospice Standards Manual* and the *Hospice Self-Assessment and Survey Guide* in 1983.

JCAH now offers the only voluntary accreditation program for hospice care for all provider types. JCAH accreditation provides consultation, review, and education to hospice programs dedicated to providing quality care and services to patients and their families.

To provide consultation on standards and survey procedures, JCAH has established an advisory committee of national experts from all hospice provider types and from all the disciplines represented on an interdisciplinary team. The committee is comprised of representatives from the National Hospice Organization, American Hospital Association, National Association of Home Care, Association of Community Cancer Centers, American Psychiatric Association, American Medical Association, National Association of Social Workers, American College of Chaplains, American Psychological Association, American Nurses' Association, and National League for Nursing, and a representative from the JCAH long-term care Professional and Technical Advisory Committee (PTAC).

Each hospice administrator must consider the benefits of voluntary accreditation, yet be alert to cost factors involved in the process. They must also consider future implications--in 1986--if we do not move ahead with the accreditation process, when determinations will be made as to continuance of the hospice benefit under Medicare.

The hospice programs that participate in JCAH's voluntary accreditation program derive many benefits from their participation. The accreditation process is an excellent tool for evaluating performance in the areas of patient/family services, continuity of care, and management. During the survey, special emphasis is placed on helping a program improve its quality of patient/family care.

Among the benefits of JCAH accreditation:

1. JCAH accreditation assists hospice programs in their efforts to provide quality care by providing the programs with an evaluation based on realistic, nationally-recognized standards.

2. JCAH staff and surveyors with experience in hospice care provide the program's staff with individualized consultation and education to aid their self-improvement efforts.

3. JCAH accreditation standards include a quality assurance process that can serve as a management control tool.

4. JCAH accreditation may facilitate the recruitment of professional staff.

5. Participating in JCAH's accreditation process motivates staff to improve services and care within a program.

6. In some instances, JCAH accreditation may facilitate reimbursement from insurance companies and other organizations and agencies.

7. JCAH accreditation demonstrates a hospice program's commitment to quality care (JCAH, 1983).

According to Barbara McCann, Director of Hospice Care Program, JCAH, problems identified through the JCAH site visits include:

- increased antagonistic relationships between attending physicians and hospice medical director

- different level of care between hospice and medicare patients

- different admission policies where patients with ALS, COPD, stroke, and cardiac are lost

- high technology home care such as hyperalimentation and chemotherapy without adequate RN training

- no conformity

- nursing is less than state of the art at home

- psychosocial services are waivering

- spiritual care is nonexistent

- no one organizational type which has proven cost effectiveness or quality.

Eleven states are now involved in the accreditation process.

In addition, there are several useful reference sources for hospice administrators with regard to hospice standards: (1) a model hospice bill prepared by NHO, called *NHO Model Legislation on Hospice*; and the *Assumptions and Principles Underlying Standards for Terminal Care*, composed by the International Work Group in Death, Dying and Bereavement (International Work Group in Death, Dying, and Bereavement, 1979; McCann, 1984).

As of May 20, 1984, only five hospices had been accredited although another four had already been surveyed and were awaiting a decision. Eight more were scheduled to be surveyed during the summer and fall of 1984 (American Hospital Association, 1984).

Interestingly, quality assurance was one of four primary areas of noncompliance. Others included: critical aspects of quality care, staffing and staff qualifications, patient/family management, and continuity of care. According to reports, some hospice programs had either no written quality assurance plan or had a plan that applies to one setting only and emphasizes problem solving rather than monitoring. Other areas mentioned that present problems for quality assurance in hospice care are as follows:

- ongoing in-service and continuing education lacked access by team members

- availability of psychosocial and spiritual services were inconsistent

- limited bereavement care training

- unclear decisions regarding the availability of IV therapy, chemotherapy, parenteral feeding, and injections in home care as well as absence of policies, procedures, and training

- unrealistic, vague, and entirely missing goals and objectives for services

- unavailability of written care plans among care settings

- lack of a resuscitation policy.

- below standard documentation of physical symptoms in home care

- notations about pain frequently occurred without mention of either the severity or the site

- lack of documentation of social work intervention making outcomes difficult to assess (McCann, 1984).

These are areas described earlier by the author as crucial to quality care in hospice programs. The accreditation process alone is an excellent mechanism for self-evaluation and evaluation by others. Hospice administrators must carefully and thoughtfully study these problem areas and seek to solve any similar weaknesses in their own program.

CERTIFICATION AS A HOSPICE PROVIDER

As discussed in Chapter 3, certification as a hospice provider is a mechanism for third-party reimbursement. The conditions of participation for certification require that a hospice must conduct an on-going, comprehensive self-assessment of the quality and appropriateness of care provided, including inpatient care and family care. The findings are used by the hospice to correct identified problems and to revise hospice policies if necessary. Hospice management must verify that the hospice has an organized quality assurance program to assess the performance of its total operation. Overall responsibility for the quality function must be assigned in writing to one individual in the hospice.

The governing body, through the hospice medical director, provides the support necessary for patient care monitoring activities and for problem identification and resolution activities. The medical staff and interdisciplinary group members implement and report on mechanisms for monitoring the quality of patient care, identify and resolve problems, and make suggestions for improving patient care. Quality assurance activities include:

- Assessment of the hospice's performance of its total operation at least once a year including all services, overall management of the hospice, and use of volunteers and other staff.

- Problem identification, assessment correction, monitoring, and documentation.

- Use of critiques by the patient's family regarding services.

- Policy implementation and monitoring of performance.

- Recommendations resulting from evaluations considered for implementation (Department of Health and Human Services, 1983).

Many state hospice networks/organizations are laying the groundwork for certification and accreditation by establishing guidelines for hospice programs for membership eligibility.* Guidelines should follow both NHO and JCAH standards to provide some basic uniformity.

Data collection and statistical information needed for hospice programs can provide insight into outcomes as a component within evaluation of quality care.

Research in quality assurance has focused on the development of quality measures, relationships between basic measurement approaches (i.e., process vs. outcome), and organizational factors associated with levels of quality. These are vital concerns since they lay the methodological foundations for understanding the nature of hospice care quality and permit the further investigation of such criticial issues as the relationship between cost and quality, access and quality, and of ethical concerns surrounding the provision or denial of clinical modalities. In spite of this extensive and growing literature, many researchers and managers concerned with improving health care quality are continually frustrated over the absence of insight regarding strategies to effect such improvement in various delivery sites. Information quantified into data and fed back to the people in an organization has some remarkable powers to facilitate organizational change, particularly when used with other interventions. If professional staff can work together to establish qualitative measures of performance, and if management can develop regular feedback mechanisms, performance can be improved (Rosen and Feigin, 1983).

As with any other element of health care coverage, the advent of more comprehensive coverage and financing is generating the pressure for "locking in" a very specific definition of hospice care and establishing standards for the delivery of high quality hospice care so that insurers can precisely define their benefit packages and be assured that they are purchasing a high quality product for their beneficiaries.

The rapid growth of hospices is creating hazards which compromise the quality of the hospice movement. Lack of control has warranted concern. Consumers cannot be guaranteed that the services they receive are truly hospice. There are vast differences between hospice programs. These variations in hospice programs are detrimental to the credibility of the movement. This hazard is not going unchallenged.

Patient outcomes, quality of care, and cost-effectiveness are terms that funders, professionals, and health care evaluators are using with increasing frequency. Cost-effectiveness is an approach to assessment of quality care which focuses on expressing the end results or outcomes of care relative to the resources consumed to produce the outcomes (costs). Cost-effectiveness brings to quality of care assessment the dimension of costs, an issue which hospice administrators must address since previously it has been either peripheral or absent from quality of care evaluation.

History suggests that quality care will improve in this era of specialization and appropriate level of care. Hospice as a specialized program can, therefore,

---

* The author served as chairman of a committee of the Pennsylvania Hospice Network to establish *Minimum Hospice Standards for Program Recognition by Pennsylvania Hospice Network.* (1984).

become a major step in delivery of quality care within our health system. Part II follows with five chapters on the varied models of hospice care.

REFERENCES

American Hospital Association. (1984). *Outreach* 5(4): entire issue.

Carr, Charles A., and Donna M. Carr. (1983). *Hospice Care Principles and Practice*. New York: Springer Publishing Company.

Department of Health and Human Services, Health Care Financing Administration. (1983). Medicare Hospice Survey Report--General Provisions.

Graham, Nancy O., ed. (1982). *Quality Assurance in Hospitals*. Rockville, MD: Aspen Systems Corporation.

International Work Group in Death, Dying, and Bereavement. (1979). Assumptions and Principles Underlying Standards for Terminal Care. *American Journal of Nursing* 79:296-297.

Joint Commission on Accreditation of Hospitals. (1983). *Hospice Standards Manual*. Chicago.

McCann, Barbara. (1984). Lecture given at Governor's Conference on an Alternative Health Care Delivery System. Hershey, PA.

Miller, James D. (Chief Executive Officer, and President, Hospice Foundation, Hospice of Pa., Inc.) (1984). Interview with author, August.

Mundinger, Mary O'Neil. (1983). *Home Care Controversy: Too Little, Too Late, Too Costly*. Rockville, MD: Aspen Systems Corporation.

Rosen, Harry M. and William Feigin. (1983). Quality Assurance and Data Feedback. *Health Care Management Review* 8(1):67-74.

Salloday, Susan A. (1984). Role Playing for Hospice Caregivers. *The American Journal of Hospice Care* 1(2):26.

PART II
HOSPICE MODELS OF CARE

Chapter 5

Hospital-Based Model

MODEL DESCRIPTION

Hospital officials with a deep commitment from administration and support from the board of directors have been successful in the implementation of a hospice program within their facility. The hospice concept requires unprecedented education of practicing professionals in the hospital as well as in the community. Hospice proponents within a hospital are fighting existing policies and procedures, and competing for funds that traditionally were used for technology and cure. External influences--the community--require collaborative relationships in addition to endorsements in order to establish a sound, quality hospice program of care within a hospital.

When the physical or psychosocial problems of the patient/family cannot be adequately addressed at home, inpatient services that recognize the privacy and dignity of the patient/family must be available. A hospice program within a hospital must evolve gradually as staff learn the new possibilities of treatment for dying patients. A hospice program must begin at the bedside of dying patients, with realistic efforts to assess their needs.

In my own experience, I have found that hospitals with a history of caring for terminal cancer patients are more inclined to accept the hospice philosophy and establish an oncology hospital-based, inpatient unit model; whereas, other hospitals without a history of specialized cancer care practice select the general hospital-based scattered-bed model. Each model will be described separately in this chapter.

JCAH Hospice Standards Manual identifies thirteen standards for inpatient services regardless of the model utilized for service provision. However, in establishing any type hospital-based model, these standards are important considerations:

I. Appropriate written policies and procedures guide the inpatient service in the delivery of hospice care.

II. An organized medical staff is responsible for the quality of hospice inpatient services provided by individuals with clinical privileges.

III.   The facility or unit where hospice inpatient services are provided maintains an organized nursing service with a sufficient number of nursing personnel to meet the level of care required by hospice patients/families.

IV.   Provision is made in the hospice inpatient setting for the privacy of patients/families.

V.   The facility or unit that provides hospice inpatient services is designed, constructed, equipped, and furnished in a manner designed to assure the physical safety of patients/families, personnel, and visitors.

VI.   The environment of the facility or unit that provides hospice inpatient services is designed, constructed, and maintained in a manner that allows for the effective delivery of clinical and personal care.

VII.   The environment of the facility or unit that provides hospice inpatient services is functionally safe and sanitary.

VIII.   The facility or unit that provides hospice inpatient services have an active infection control program.

IX.   The facility or unit that provides hospice inpatient services meets the nutritional and special dietary needs of patients.

X.   The facility or unit that provides hospice inpatient services meets the pharmaceutical needs of patients.

XI.   The facility or unit that provides hospice inpatient services provides, or has delineated access to, radiology services.

XII.   The facility or unit that provides hospice inpatient services provides, or has delineated access to, pathology and laboratory services in accordance with the needs of the patients, the size of the facility or unit, the services offered, and the resources available in the community.

XIII.   The facility or unit that provides hospice inpatient services provides, or has delineated access to, emergency services. (JCAH, 1983).

A TYPICAL ONCOLOGY HOSPITAL-BASED INPATIENT HOSPICE

Formal and Informal Structure

A typical inpatient unit is found within a hospital in a location conducive to a homelike environment but close to the chapel, outdoors, and other crucial areas with eight to ten discrete beds.

One New York State inpatient unit's organizational structure is under the aegis of Daughters of Charity, a religious order of the Roman Catholic Church. The hospice unit consists of ten beds within a facility of over 300 beds which serves as a cancer center for a five-county area providing oncology and radiation services as well as a community education program on cancer care and death and dying.

Units familiar to the author initiate efforts by their palliative care team visiting other similar hospice programs such as Royal Victoria in Montreal and St. Christopher's in England to gather information on the hospice philosophy and provision of care. Simultaneously or shortly thereafter, a feasibility study conducted by the facility provides necessary information for planning and acquisition of a certificate of need if required.

The inpatient hospice coordinates with the hospital board of trustees through a hospice advisory board, an autonomous group with a large membership.* This group meets monthly for planning and evaluation and consists of representation from the hospital board of trustees, finance committee, evaluation committee, home care committee, pastoral care committee, bereavement committee, medical-nursing committee, and public relations committee.

Direct observations during tours of facilities revealed that the hospice inpatient facility is often located near the chapel in the hospital. A living room, dining room, activities room, and small kitchen are provided for the comfort of the family. The hospice unit differs from the remainder of the hospital in its home-like environment including the absence of visitor restrictions, no uniforms worn by staff, permission for pets and children to visit, the ability for patient and family to prepare food, and the availability of overnight accommodations. Inpatient beds are utilized when symptoms cannot be controlled at home, in the absence of a primary caregiver, or when the primary care person needs a rest. This unit supplements the coordinated home care program when the patient needs hospitalization.

The inpatient hospice may contract with a county health department, local public health nursing agency, or visiting nurse association for provision of home care from 9 a.m. to 5 p.m. Monday through Friday and on call Saturday and Sunday from 8 a.m. to 12 noon. For the remainder of the time, coverage is accomplished by the inpatient unit team.

Program Components

Program components within a hospital-based discrete unit include inpatient hospice care, coordinated home care, bereavement counseling, and education.

Their philosophy is that death is a universal fact of life and whether or not it is accompanied by disease, dying is a normal process. The stated belief of the board of trustees is that every person is entitled to participate fully in this part of life in order to prepare for death in a way that is personally satisfying. Hospice, as an option in the medical care system, exists not to postpone death but to help the patient and family live as fully as possible with special skills and therapies.

---

* One hospice advisory board consists of sixty members.

During administrative interviews in one facility this philosophy was further explained as follows:

Death is not denied but life is affirmed and lived until death comes. We are all dependent on one another, therefore, it is crucial, in the last few months of life, to help develop a caring community that can provide comprehensive services to patients and their families.

According to patient care manuals, a discrete hospice unit seeks to provide care for the terminally ill that allows the patient to maintain dignity through the control of pain, the offer of specialized nursing care appropriate for the patient, and provision of psychological support for the patient and family as they together adapt to the implications of an ending life. An inpatient hospice unit provides:

- Care and comfort.

- Symptom control and physical care in home with inpatient care provided when caregivers need a rest or symptoms cannot be controlled.

- Maximum quality of remaining life while moving the family toward a quiet resolution of impending death. Each patient is treated as a unique individual with specialized needs.

- Skilled care without sacrificing companionship of the family. A plan is designed to strengthen and sustain family relationships and allow family to maintain responsibility for care within coping capabilities in a community of caring persons who support one another.

- Care to maximum comfort while remaining cognizant of the fact that the patient's status may change, requiring an alternative level of care.

- A goal to relieve all total pain (physical, spiritual, psychosocial, financial).

- High staff/patient ratio that will allow time for interdisciplinary care planning, an unhurried approach to care, time for listening and supporting, and time to meet educational responsibilities.

- A quality assurance program through the hospital quality assurance person who works with the hospice staff to develop evaluation procedures for nursing in cooperation with the hospital's evaluation coordinator.

Hospice home care services contracted from community differ from the traditional home care in that more time (daily from two to four hours as compared to three hours weekly by the traditional public health nurse) is spent in the home with the patient/family, and funeral preparations and bereavement counseling are included as a component of their visits.

Bereavement coordination may be done initially by a registered nurse voluntarily on a part-time basis. However, as a program progresses, there is the increasing need for a full-time bereavement coordinator.

The inpatient-based hospice is designed for care of patients with limited life expectancy (a terminal illness with a prognosis of weeks or months). Emphasis is placed upon improving the quality of life for the patient and family during the advanced stages of disease. The goals are to allow the patient to live at home in his or her customary environment as long as appropriate and to support the family in caring for the patient. Part of this support is the inpatient facility where patients can be treated for alleviation of the symptoms, especially pain, of advanced-stage disease. Hospice care at all times aims at improving the quality of life during the final stages for the patient/family.

A review of referral procedures revealed that initial contact with the hospice program may be made by a physician, patient, family member, friend, or outside agency to the hospice director of patient family services. At that time, the hospice concept is explained and the personal physician is then contacted for recommendations. After a social, nursing, and medical evaluation, the hospice team and personal physician decide upon the appropriateness of admission. Admission criteria are:

- The physician has determined that aggressive treatment to modify the course of disease is no longer suitable. Life expectancy is in terms of weeks or months, not years.

- The patient requires treatment of symptoms, especially pain, and/or emotional, spiritual, or social support.

- The patient, family, and physician, where involved, agree to the admission.

- Responsible persons must be available to work with the hospice team in caring for the patient when at home.

Inpatient-based hospice services include:

- social work assessment and consultation

- skilled nursing care at home

- inpatient hospice facility

- medical consultation

- volunteer services

- dietary consultation

- pastoral care

- individual and group bereavement support

- availability by telephone twenty-four hours a day, seven days a week.

One statistical report showed that out of 155 patient/families, 40 percent were female and 60 percent were male. One hundred and thirty six have died. These 136 patients generated 3,566.5 patient days. Of these, 1,562.5 were in the inpatient part of hospice. Thus, patients averaged approximately 11.5 days on the unit. Two thousand two hundred fifty-two patient days on home care were generated or 16.5 on average. One hundred fifty-two days were spent in contact with the hospice program while the patient remained in some institution, usually a hospital or a nursing home, outside of the hospice. Thus, the average length of stay on the program was approximately twenty-nine days. Cancer of the lung is the most common cause of death followed by cancer of the breast and colon.

The inpatient unit has an ongoing educational program for board members, volunteers, staff, patient/family, and community. All hospital staff in all the hospitals in the geographic area and all public health nurses are specially trained in hospice care by the inpatient hospice staff through educational seminars. Consultation services are also provided to area hospitals. The educational meeting calendar includes weekly admission team conferences, weekly patient care team conferences, weekly patient conferences with the psychologist, weekly support and relaxation sessions with a psychologist for staff, monthly bereavement conferences for staff and families, and biweekly nursing staff meetings to facilitate communications between shifts and discuss projects in which they are involved. A review of one educational calendar showed that ongoing in-service education topics include stress, family and terminal care, pain control, bereavement, and legal aspects. Audio-visual tapes are always available for patients, families, and children in the living room of the inpatient unit as observed during the site visit. Community presentations are made by staff upon request and frequently occur weekly. Staff attend workshops and educational conferences held by administration on a monthly basis as noted in summaries of meetings with the goal of assisting to maintain and improve the quality of the hospice program.

A typical patient's day in the inpatient hospice unit at a hospital is spent in various rooms within the unit, that is, living room area, dining or conference room, kitchen and patient room, with team members mingling throughout the day. A tour of one unit revealed various patients with multiple needs. During an interview with the director of family services, the hospice team was called upon to assist in the transfer of a patient from his reclining chair to his bed requiring several people to participate in lifting, including the volunteer, nurses, social worker, and director. Patients were seen throughout the day by the director, professional nurses, licensed practical nurses, aides, hospital dietician, social worker, clergy, and volunteers. Family members were observed preparing food in a small kitchen for a patient who desired a special dish and home cooking. Families are allowed to bring in special food. However, the hospital provides food for the families to prepare if they wish. In the living room a patient was observed sitting in a reclining chair watching television and conversing with his family members. A five-year-old grandson was sitting in one section of the living room with a volunteer reviewing an audio-visual presentation for children on death and dying. A family was holding a birthday party in another room in the unit which was set up as a conference or dining room. They had birthday cake and ice cream to celebrate an elderly patient's birthday.

A new patient was seen wheeled in a bed down the hall from another department of the hospital with three family members following closely alongside and hospice staff joining as they proceeded to a private room for the patient within the unit. The director of family services quickly brought everyone together (hospice staff, patient, and family) introducing each team member and explaining their role in patient care during their stay in the inpatient unit.

In another area, family and staff were observed surrounding a patient's bed in a private room while the patient was in his final stage of life.

Patients are encouraged to attend the unit for special events and occasions. One patient who wished to go on a fishing trip and attend a family reunion was able to do so because the hospice staff arranged to borrow a van from a local car dealer and volunteered to take him, in his bed, with their assistance for the weekend. He recounted that he saw relatives he hadn't seen in some time and was able to talk with each of them as they greeted him at the reunion.

Staffing Patterns

The inpatient hospice unit is physician-directed and nurse-coordinated. The hospice unit is often administered by a designated hospice administrator formally from the hospital.

The inpatient unit hospice team may consist of five registered nurses, two licensed practical nurses, two health aides, a director of patient/family services who is a registered nurse, medical director, social worker, director of volunteers, a clinical psychologist, pastoral care coordinator, dietician, and psychiatric consultant for ten beds.

In a policy statement entitled "Role of Public Health Nurses and Inpatient Nurses Re: Hospice Home Care Patients," the role of the public health nurses (PHNs) and inpatient nurses can be clearly defined. PHNs manage all aspects of home care under supervision of the patient's physician. All home care patients are followed by the inpatient unit team. A twenty-four hour telephone line is available in addition to home visits from various team members (physician, nursing, social worker, pastoral care, volunteers). Home care patients are followed by the public health department, the hospice's community team member. According to a professional nurse coordinator, communication between the public health liaison nurse and home care nurse occurs daily as needed on an informal basis and formally every week. They evaluate the ability of the hospice team to fully meet the patient's needs at home and they reassess the patient and/or family situation continually. Weekly conferences are held at the hospital inpatient unit at which time the public health liaison nurse confers with the other team members regarding patient's condition, family's condition, problems, highlights, suggestions, and advice. Daily contact is also made regarding particular problems between the designated PHN liaison person and inpatient nurse or director of patient/family services who correlate information gathered and relay with one phone call to provide consistency.

Resources Available

According to one job description the director of volunteers, who holds a bachelor of science degree in human services, selects and educates volunteers in the hospice concept and coordinates the volunteer activities of the hospice. Volunteers are involved in patient visitation and support of the family, and assist in all aspects of the hospice program. In a monthly training program for new volunteers, over eighty were trained from the end of 1979 to 1981. According to the written program summary, the educational program allows the trainee to explore his own feelings about death, and share those feelings with others. The program also consists of lectures on cancer, pain control, aging, and the grief-stricken family.

Funding Sources

Under the Hevesi-Farley Law, established in New York state in 1978, hospice demonstration programs were established to care for the medical and emotional needs of the terminally ill and their families.

According to one hospice administrator, the cost of hospice care in the hospital to the patient/family is the same as care in other places in the hospital. Billing is handled in the same manner. Since prolonged illness often creates monetary concern for the family, the hospice social worker assists the family in planning its finances during this period. Third-party reimbursement for skilled home care is handled by the organization providing home care services through a written contract; the inpatient hospice is unable to become a certified home health agency in some states due to state certificate-of-need regulations. In approaching cost, the inpatient hospice unit hopes to decrease the length of a hospital stay and decrease the number of needless multiple tests and procedures ordered by physicians to demonstrate cost-saving factors for hospice care.

A TYPICAL GENERAL HOSPITAL-BASED SCATTERED-BED MODEL

Formal and Informal Structure

A typical scattered-bed hospice program comprises ten to twelve scattered beds throughout a large not-for-profit community hospital serving 250,000 residents of a suburban community. A feasibility study in that county shows 264 residents of the hospital's service area died from cancer during the year the hospice program was started.

In programs familiar to the author, services are provided by the cooperative efforts of a nursing corporation, a visiting nurse association, and the hospital. One entire program was sparked by a letter from a minister regarding his interest and commitment. During an interview the nurse coordinator related that a highly motivated and skilled group of trustees, doctors, nurses, clergy, and volunteers were appointed to a hospice advisory committee for the purpose of developing and establishing the program. In less than a year, they created an innovative program to help ease the ordeal for the increasing number of families who must deal with terminal cancer. According to a written description of committees, the hospice advisory committee acts as a liaison between the hospital and the two cooperating agencies, promotes public relations, educates paid and volunteer caregivers and the lay community, and serves in a general advisory capacity to the program. The board of trustees of the hospital oversees the program through the hospice administrator who is also a member of the management staff to the hospital and has the decision-making authority for expenditures of all hospice funds committed by the hospital.

Because of the lengthy process involved in filing for certificate of need in some states, a hospice may become a coordinated program rather than a new service. If possible, hospice patients are admitted to the oncology unit where registered nurses are trained in hospice care; however, if the "scattered" bed is elsewhere in the hospital, the hospice team works directly with the floor staff. A written brochure for hospice patients states that visiting hours are unlimited-- anytime of day or night, any number of visitors, any age and pets are allowed with discretion. All hospice patients have private rooms.

Program Components

Proponents of the hospice program at one scattered-bed hospital have believed for a long time that there was a better way to help people who were dying, and to provide doctors with an immediate means of engaging a team of people whose training and expertise--and philosophy of love and caring--could ease the pain for both patient and family. While there has been a great deal of talk in death-and-dying circles about emotional problems, there has been far too little concern about the patient's physical comfort. Thus, for the hospital-based scattered-bed hospice program, the most important part of hospice care is symptom control. One patient care coordinator expressed the following philosophy:

> Those who are caring for the dying are concerned about controlling pain, smoothing sheets, and sitting up at night. A certain amount of role-blending is necessary to ensure the patient's comfort at all times. In hospice, there is never a time when "nothing more can be done." Granted some people want every dollop of life that medical technology can provide . . . no matter how severe the physical or emotional suffering.

But more and more people are concerned about increasing the quality of the last days of life.

An inpatient hospice program with scattered beds also includes a coordinated home care component, a bereavement program, and an educational program. The objectives are to meet the needs of the terminally ill patients that have not been met under previous systems of health care in their communities. Hospice care ensures that the quality of life remaining is as comfortable and satisfying as possible with the direction of treatment and care toward symptom control. The program is family-oriented, providing palliative and supportive care to the patient and supportive care to the family including physical, emotional, spiritual, social, and economic considerations during the final stages of life and in their bereavement period following. Hospital and home care are coordinated to provide a twenty-four hour continuity of care and purpose.

It is interesting to note that in one scattered-bed program half of the referrals are made to the program by the community, for example patients and family, and/or the over sixty primary physicians who participate in hospice, half of whom are from the hospital. According to a review of the written referral process, patient/families referred to the program who do not meet the eligibility criteria are not abandoned but rather alternatives are sought by referral to other community resources.

Criteria for admission to the hospital scattered-bed hospice program are typically:

- The hospice patient should live within the geographic area serviced by the hospital and the home care agencies.

- The personal physician should agree with the hospice philosophy and procedures are aimed to relieve symptoms of disease rather than give active treatment for cure.

- Terminal care with a three to six month life expectancy.

- A primary caregiver who will take the responsibility for care of the hospice patient should be in the home. The primary caregiver may be a family member, friend, or paid companion who has agreed to assume primary responsibility.

Statistics show that this type model has a caseload of twenty-five patients with 50 percent female and 50 percent male. Initially the length of stay in one program was thirteen days, six months later it was twenty-nine days, and now it is thirty-six days. At the onset of the program, 75 percent of the patients died in the hospital, now 61 percent die at home. Lung cancer is the most common cause of death, followed by breast and colon.

A comprehensive educational program is carried out for volunteers, hospice staff and VNA professional nurses regarding hospice care and bereavement and then every other month on an on-going basis. Presentations are given to community groups. In addition, the hospital's development director is responsible for a presentation which is given for organizations, corporations, and individuals interested in helping to fund hospice. Monthly bereavement rap sessions are held as well as monthly volunteer rap sessions. According to a summary of volunteer activities in one program, fifty-five volunteers have participated in training sessions of two hours a week for twelve weeks duration.

In the formal statement on the agency bereavement program, the hospice program is described as a coordination of resources in order to meet the physical, emotional, spiritual, social, and economic needs during the final stages of life, and the bereavement period following. The hospice's bereavement program consists of the family's preparation for the death of a patient, attendance at the time of death, aid and support in making the necessary decisions regarding funerals, and attendance at the funeral. It also provides contact with the family after death and referrals to counseling programs if necessary.

Since hospice patients are scattered throughout the hospital, the author did not observe hospice inpatients as separate from other patients. Family members were observed visiting the hospice offices which are in a separate section of the hospitals to talk with staff about their problems. A patient care coordinator stated that hospice team members visit patients on the floors initially for assessment and then according to need. Numerous telephone contacts were heard between home patients and staff from the hospice offices during a site visit by the author. By policy, the members of one scattered-bed team are authorized to make rounds of the hospital with floor staff to look for patients who ought to be considered for the hospice program. Such explorations are usually made by a social worker, a nurse from home care, and the nurse who heads the hospice team. (Rossman, 1979).

Staffing Patterns

The hospice team may consist of the patient care coordinator (a registered professional nurse), a full-time secretary, a part-time medical director, a consultant pharmacist, a half-time social worker, a psychologist with a doctoral degree in thanatology, and a director of volunteers (a registered professional nurse) working two-thirds time. One professional nurse coordinator states that services are provided by the hospice staff team, visiting nurse association (VNA) nurses, and VNA hospice coordinators. One visiting nurse agency has approximately ten registered professional nurses and the second VNA has fifteen. Three to four professional nurses from each VNA are carrying hospice patients and share twenty-four hour call. Hospice nurses from the VNAs are expected to spend more time in the homes in comparison to the traditional home care visits and also to assist in funeral arrangements unlike the routine home care visits.

In an interview, the patient care coordinator outlined staff responsibilities as follows: assessment, planning, implementation, coordination, evaluation, reassessment, communication, and recording of the hospice program for each patient/family in connection with the orders of the primary physician and the guidelines set by the medical director. The patient care coordinator utilizes all community resources within the three agencies and, in addition to them, recommends further development of resources as experience proves their necessity for patient care. The patient care coordinator is also responsible for administrative functions which include staff development and evaluation, budget management, data recording, and other relevant functions. The medical social worker does psychosocial and financial counseling. The director of volunteers is responsible for the selection, education, and evaluation of volunteers. The medical director of the hospice program is a member of the staff of the hospital and a member of the hospice advisory committee whose responsibility is to develop and uphold the general concepts of hospice care. The medical director serves as a hospice consultant to the medical staff of the three agencies and the patient's primary physician and acts as an advisor and resource person for the patient care coordinator and other members of the hospice team. The clergy are recognized as a part of the hospice team.

Resources Available

The volunteers, sometimes called hospice assistants, are an integral part of the support system. A written description of volunteer services may state that they offer support and companionship for patients and their families with specific emphasis on functions such as taking the children of a patient out on a recreational trip, doing errands, shopping, doing jobs around the home, providing transportation, or just sitting with a patient when appropriate. Volunteer support and other services are provided through funding and donations at no cost to the hospice patient and/or family.

Typical community agencies for coordination are Cancer Care, American Cancer Society, Red Cross for transportation, Family Counseling Service, and Meals on Wheels.

Funding Sources

A review of cost revealed that the cost of the time spent by a hospice patient in a scattered-bed unit at the hospital as a hospice inpatient is the same as traditional care. Skilled home care provided to a hospice patient is covered through the existing third-party reimbursement by the contracted home care agencies. Any noncovered hospice home care costs are then billed to the hospital-based scattered-bed hospice program.

Funding resources may come from large donations from supportive businesses and large donations from oncology families. Gifts are also received from estates, corporations, churches, and families and friends of patients. The parent hospital contributes a large annual sum from fundraising efforts. A speakers' bureau and memorials also provide donations. A hospice program brochure states that skilled nursing services are reimbursed through third-party payers or on a sliding scale according to the ability to pay. No person is ever refused necessary care due to inability to pay.

ADVANTAGES AND DISADVANTAGES

Hospital-based programs in general tend to ease the problems of the curative-palliative interface. Transition from one approach to the other is usually relatively smooth in such programs. Anti-tumor therapy for palliative purposes is more convenient in an acute general hospital. Hospitals can also make available to the patient other sophisticated forms of care which can contribute to palliation. Naturally, although the hospice patient is not subjected to many tests or treatments, there are times when the easy availability of an X-ray or an intramedullary nail can be most helpful in making a patient comfortable. In addition, one of the major advantages of the hospital-based program is the relatively ready availability of expert specialized team individuals. The inpatient discrete unit has addressed numerous hospice problems for solution and, by tradition, their oncology hospital-based inpatient unit suits hospice. The director of social services at a rural Pennsylvania hospital with a hospital-based hospice program with scattered beds declares that the key to their success is an administrator committed to hospice principles since reimbursement is the same as acute care.

There is another advantage to a hospital-based unit. Much of what is generic to hospice care can be of benefit to patients who are not terminally ill. Hospice principles, may very well influence other types of health care in hospital-based units. As stated by Zimmerman (1981), one of the advantages of the freestanding model has been the presumed inability of hospitals to be sufficiently flexible in implementation of policies to make hospice care workable. Hospitals are seen as cold, impersonal, and rigid. To the contrary, he claims his Church Hospital Hospice Care Program's experience has been that the same hospital is quite capable of providing the highest quality of curative medicine and top-flight care for the terminally ill.

The inpatient discrete unit setting has the advantage of being able to maintain control of their program through a specialized care team who focus on expert palliative care with unlimited resources within their institution. In hospitals with a history of providing care to terminal cancer patients, hospice has commitment from the hospital board of directors and administration who supports them in program development and provision of services. Furthermore, the history of the role of the hospital in their specialized care of the terminally ill provides a smooth transition from curative to palliative care. A medical director who specializes in hospice care permits desirable features of hospice care to cross-fertilize general medical care in their institution. Traditional hospital policies and practice acts hinder a uniform approach to a specialized type of terminal care--hence the advantage of a separate unit with specific policies and procedures in rendering hospice care under the certification of the hospice medical director, a recommended criterion for admission to the unit. A number of individual primary physicians makes it more difficult to assume hospice standards of care because of the lack of control on medical care practice. Also acute care training of personnel has run counter to that needed for hospice care.

The response of one family member in the hospital based inpatient unit was:

> I would like to add my own thoughts about the hospice program. Although my husband has not as yet needed to go into the hospice unit--the moral support and just knowing that when he needs to use the service--it is there--a warm caring place for his last days is a great relief. . .

From my own experience and research, I have concluded that the hospital-based inpatient unit appears to be more effective than the scattered-bed model in providing quality care. Administrative and supervisory control in one geographic area in the hospital enables the hospice staff to function completely as a team in administering direct care themselves; for example, they are able to care for several patients at one time and utilize standard guidelines for giving pain medication which they are responsible for implementing and monitoring. In the scattered-bed situation, the educational process and turnover of floor staff presents a problem in assuring use of the hospice concept and philosophy.

Both types of hospital inpatient programs have the advantage over other hospice models of unlimited resources within their institution allowing an effective application of the interdisciplinary care team. Their major advantage is a committed hospital administrator who promotes their hospice program within the community, supports their needs, and assists with problems as they arise. Each inpatient hospital-based model is cost-effective utilizing the existing reimbursement system. This is an advantage in that the funding mechanism is not interrupted--unlike most freestanding models that lack continued funding.

A major disadvantage of a scattered-bed model is that the hospice team does not function in a specific unit for direct care; patients are dispersed in widely separated areas throughout the hospital. The hospice team role changes and becomes a symptom support control team. A diametrically opposed philosophy of acute and palliative care exists within hospital administration. The hospital environment may be inflexible and frightening as well as impersonal. In a scattered-bed model the *cohesive impact* of a hospice team is lessened, and hospice becomes a consultative service. It becomes very difficult for every staff member to be well-educated and experienced in hospice protocol, especially in the area of pain and medication around the clock. The educational component within the scattered-bed model becomes an endless process. Nevertheless, the institution-based models actually practice administration of pain medication around the clock.

Another difficulty is coordinating the home care program which tends to limit control of services provided even though a formal agreement exists between the scattered-bed hospice program and the local home care agencies, or even a hospital's own home care program and a discrete unit. This liaison for home care presents a difficult management problem. Medical record keeping, orientation of home health staff, and effective and timely communication of patient care plans are more complicated.

In addition, a disadvantage of some inpatient discrete unit hospice programs is their inability, due to certificate of need such as in New York and New Jersey, to provide their own home health care services. In order to assure continuity of care a sophisticated liaison program is followed requiring very close monitoring. Continuity of care is not a soundly-based practice with coordination in the community because formal contracts are not always feasible.

To summarize, advantages of the hospital-based models include:

- An administrative team representing various disciplines

- Unlimited resources within the overall institutional setting

- Cross-fertilization of hospice care with general medical care

- Cost-effectiveness utilizing existing reimbursement system

Disadvantages include:

- Administrator is also responsible for other programs which are complex and changing

- Diametrically opposed philosophies of acute and palliative care within hospital administration

- Continuity soundly-based practice with coordination in the community

QUALITY AND THE HOSPITAL-BASED MODEL

Discrete Unit

The discrete inpatient unit provides an environment in which almost two-thirds of the criteria for quality care were met. Those criteria involving direct patient care which were met were provision of twenty-four hour services, treatment of the patient/family as a unit of care, the coordination of patient/family services, palliative care, and flexibility and continuity in providing care.

Pain control, according to the hospice standard of administration of pain medication around the clock, was met in 68 percent of the patients surveyed by the author. One physician advocates a double dose of pain medication at hour of sleep and omitting the 2 a.m. dose which is most effective in allowing patients to sleep through the night.* It appears that the single most common reason for admission to inpatient status is inadequate pain control. Although patients can be managed on very high doses of narcotics at home, the titration process by which the optimal pattern of narcotic administration is achieved requires close observation and frequent dosage change which are difficult to execute outside the hospital. Since fear of additional pain is an important symptom in the terminally ill, the institution-based programs found that use of analgesics on an as-needed basis plays little role in the management of chronic pain. Analgesic medication must be given on a regular basis, as any psychological and social problems can aggravate physical symptoms.

Pastoral care services were provided for 53 percent of the patients. The use of the extended hospice care team was limited since 50 percent of the patients received services from the traditional team. There may be a relationship between the amount of pastoral care, team involvement, and effective pain control. The relationship between pastoral services and pain control variables can be noted in the hospital-based inpatient unit. Pain, discomfort, and anxiety are often compounded with physical, mental, social, and spiritual elements; therefore, use of the interdisciplinary team is essential. Because many factors are involved in pain perception, a successful approach to pain requires knowledge and counseling of all the elements involved in the patient's situation requiring the expertise of the various team members including clergy.

Adequate support in coping with problems through use of the hospice team for the emotional, social, and spiritual counseling which relates directly to data results in pain control from medical record audit can greatly simplify the management of physical symptoms.

One could speculate that the institution-based hospice sites advocates the practice of pain medication around the clock due to the support and closer supervision and assessment by the professional and also that hospice patients become inpatients at a point of high pain levels.

A relationship may also exist between direct hospice administration and the fulfillment of the other quality criteria. Direct administration controls the quality of care provided through twenty-four hour service, volunteer services, bereavement services, and commitment to the patient/family as a unit of care.

Indirect care criteria met were use of a separate administrator, the existing reimbursement system, and an educational program.

---

* The brompton cocktail--a mixture of morphine sulfate and cocaine in a vehicle of alcohol, syrup and chloroform water--was first used for control of chronic pain in hospices throughout England, Canada, and the United States. There is no advantage in the brompton cocktail when compared to a simple solution of morphine sulfate alone or in a vehicle, e.g., cherry syrup or aromatic elixir. The use of cocaine, alcohol, and chloroform water add nothing to the drug therapy and should be discouraged. The brompton cocktail is no longer used. Morphine sulfate is probably the single most effective agent for control of chronic pain.

Due to admission policy and strict hospice philosophy, the discrete inpatient unit does not practice active antitumor therapy and use of X-rays and diagnostic studies. The admission criterion reads:

Never acceptable is active chemotherapy (ex: 20.V. drugs), blood and platelet therapy, and active radiation for prolongation of life.

The lack of a formal evaluation program may relate to limited use of the extended interdisciplinary team. An evaluation program may assist staff in doing a more in-depth and comprehensive patient/family care assessment resulting in a need for additional team components.

In the hospice models, concern for human beings transcends traditional professional roles and prerogatives; teamwork blends a variety of insights and skills of volunteers, professionals, and nonprofessionals. A team approach can draw upon professional expertise from a variety of fields in order to resolve difficulties. Furthermore, medical record audit showed that patients are highly individual in their ability to relate to other people; therefore, the availability of many team members provides the opportunity for support from a number of sources. It is not uncommon for the most important emotional support to come from a nonprofessional member of the team. An important feature of the interdisciplinary hospice team is the lack of sharp distinction between the functions of the various team members. Although each has his area of expertise and primary responsibility, each should seek to be alert to the needs of the patient in other areas and all should share in providing psychological and emotional support to the patient and family.

The hospital-based inpatient unit utilized health aides less frequently than the scattered-bed site. This appears to depend on the custom or policy of the parent institution. The health aide, a paraprofessional team member, assists the nurse in providing personal care services to the patient. Each hospital has different practices regarding variations in staffing. The psychologist or psychiatrist and physical therapist were rarely used as part of the team. Local circumstances may determine the utilization of various disciplines as to availability of qualified professionals in hospice care. Each hospice group designs its own approach and chooses the most appropriate staff with expertise in hospice care. Psychiatrists with the requisite skill are not available to all hospice groups.

Physical therapy for hospice patients has a somewhat different orientation; therefore, not all physical therapists are suited to this type of work. The goals of the physical therapist are to help the terminally ill patient adapt to his physical limitations and to permit him to function at his highest possible physical level. Physical therapists are also involved with pain control, such as use of the Transcutaneous Electrical Nerve Stimulation (TENS). The prime requirements are a special interest in working with the terminally ill, the ability to work cooperatively with the interdisciplinary team, adaptability, some knowledge of the issues of death, dying, and grief, and an understanding of and agreement with hospice care principles. Physical therapists are difficult to recruit in some geographic areas according to hospice directors. Also physicians are not educated on how to utilize the services of a physical therapist with their terminal patients.

The approach to management of the terminally ill patient must be individualized. The patient with a substantial life expectancy may be helped by better nutrition, whereas this consideration becomes irrelevant for the patient with a very limited life expectancy. Again, physicians are not always accustomed to writing specific orders for a nutrition consultation. Physicians do depend on nurses to handle the nutritional aspects of care. Patients in home care traditionally look to the nurse for nutritional guidance.

For work with home care patients, it is often helpful for a hospice program to involve at least one private pharmacy outside the hospital. According to medical record audit, in hospice care, drugs are used both in conventional and unconventional fashions and dosages, particularly in pain relief. It is important that the hospital or local pharmacy staff be conversant with principles of hospice care since high dose morphine solution, dilaudid suppositories, and artificial saliva are seldom used in nonhospice patients. The hospital-based models utilize the hospital pharmacist, unlike a community-based model program which has a private pharmacist as a volunteer consultant on the professional advisory committee. Use of a pharmacist as a paid staff team component is not essential since private and hospital pharmacists are accessible when needed for consultation purposes.

Scattered Beds

A scattered-bed unit site within a hospital provides a twenty-four hour service, commitment to the patient/family as a unit of care, a coordination for patient/family services, and provision of bereavement services. Half of the patients in the scattered-bed program received services from the extended hospice team and volunteer component with minimal pastoral care services--10 percent of the patients. The pain control criterion was met in half of the patients. This, too, shows a relationship between use of the team, especially clergy, in pain control.

With regard to direct care criteria not carried out: there were no formal education and evaluation programs. Again, as in the discrete unit, this may be related to limited use of the team component. Unlike the discrete unit, the scattered-bed unit does not have a separate administrator, but a coordinator for the hospice program which may affect proper use of all team members.

Administrative Considerations

The hospital-based models do have a distinct parent organization which not only provides administration but also funding support for their hospice program.

Patient characteristics will vary geographically and also according to admission criteria. The level of the patients' acute conditions will determine staffing needs. State licensure requirements state a variety of staffing ratios. Those hospice patients with a very poor prognosis are acute patients with multiple pathologies, multiple symptoms, compromised metabolic processes, and complex treatment plans. Management of pain and other symptoms requires constant assessment, diagnosis, and titration of medications and other treatments. Many patients requiring hospice inpatient care have complicated wounds, severe decubitus ulcers, multiple draining fistulae which involve frequent irrigations, and dressing changes and ostomy care. Multiple diagnoses provide a complexity of problems from other chronic medical illnesses such as cardiac, renal, and pulmonary disease, and diabetes aggravated by a primary diagnosis of cancer. Moreover, the emotional complications intensify a twenty-four hour need for quality nursing care. Thus, the type of patient requiring a higher level of care is found in a hospice inpatient model where the staffing pattern required resembles a medical-surgical intensive care unit. As stated by one physician, hospice inpatient care is not a "soft option." It is not a low-level service (Johnson-Hurzeber, Rosemary, Evelyn Barnum, and John Abbott). Hospice inpatient care is labor intensive, particularly in the medical and nursing area; however, it requires social work staff, arts and pastoral care staff, pharmacy staff, volunteer staff, counselors, and consultants. The worth of human interaction is emphasized, rather than the increasingly technical environment.

Most importantly, development of the hospice setting within a hospital must project a mood and purpose conducive to quality hospice care. "Hospice imperative" includes comfort for living activities, accommodations for family participation, an atmosphere which conveys a message, and privacy for intimacy and for grieving. Staff must understand the community and must be selected on the basis of flexibility, outside interests, and spiritual development in addition to professional credentials.

Effective integration of home and inpatient treatment programs provides for administrative efficiency, cost savings, and patient/family confidence. The question remains: Is this possible within a hospital-based model? Chapter 6 describes the home care model as a possibility for model selection.

REFERENCES

Johnson-Hurzeler, Rosemary, Evelyn Barnum, and John Abbott. (1983). Hospice: The Beginning or The End?: The Impact of TEFRA on Hospice Care In The United States. *University of Bridgeport Law Review* (1):69-105.

Joint Commission on Accreditation of Hospitals. (1983). *Hospice Standards Manual*. Chicago.

Rossman, Parker. (1979). *Hospice.* New York: Fawcett Columbine.

Zimmerman, Jack M. (1981). *Hospice: Complete Care for the Terminally Ill.* Baltimore-Munich: Urban and Schwarzenberg.

Chapter 6

Home Care Model

Traditional home health agencies such as fifty-year-old (or more) visiting nurse associations have been providing home care to cancer patients for years. With this experience one might expect that this model would be ideal for a hospice setting. Home health agency hospice programs provide care either through an identified hospice team or as a specialty service where all staff provide care to identified hospice patients with similar informal arrangements for inpatient care.

A home care agency that has expanded into a hospice does not automatically insure quality of care for patients and may also run the risk of exceeding the family's physical, emotional, and financial limits. To minimize these risks, home care must include adequate support services, aimed at the needs of patients and caregivers (Gold, 1983). The home may become a center where family or friends can provide elements of care including medications, exercise, diet, treatments, and nursing procedures which have been taught by the hospice team. Medications can be regulated to maintain the patient's alertness even though symptoms and pain are controlled. The hospice team assesses the patient's and family's level of knowledge, abilities, and goals in order to facilitate plans for home care. The level of pain, whether physical, psychological, spiritual, or social, is often related to the ability of the family to deal with stress and disturbed equilibrium. Hospice staff, unlike the traditional home health agency staff, are accessible twenty-four hours a day to talk with or help the family group.

A TYPICAL HOME CARE MODEL

Formal and Informal Structure

In home care models I am familiar with, a hospice program becomes a component of a voluntary nonprofit public health nursing agency that traditionally provides nursing services, medical social services, therapy services (occupational, speech, and physical), chore service, homemaker/home health aide service, and sick room equipment to serve the needs of residents of the county. The traditional home health agency is frequently an accredited member of the National Council of Homemaker/Home Health Aide Service, Inc., is certified for Medicare reimbursement as a home health agency, and is a member of the United Way.

As a formal independent private community organization governed by a voluntary board of directors, services are coordinated with hospitals and social service agencies in the community on an informal basis and mainly for referrals. These informal relationships exist to facilitate sources of service support for home care patients.

In the home care models researched by this author, a community steering committee approached the home care agency board of directors regarding the implementation of a hospice program as a component of the existing agency. Based on concern for the dying patient and his family in their communities, physicians, clergy, and the hospitals joined forces in support of the development of a palliative home care program as an extension of the traditional home health agency (VNA) with the knowledge that hospice services in the United States focus on home care.

Program Components

Hospice home care programs have been developed around the philosophy that care for the dying patient must be coordinated under medical direction; the dying patient should end his day with less stress than is often endured; pain and symptoms can be reduced or eliminated; and the family has a need for support at the time of death and beyond. [Hospice program supporters believe that the hospice concept offers an alternative to the traditional way of responding to death by delaying it as long as possible--regardless of the price.] Thus many terminally ill patients with chronic, degenerative disease stay for an extended period on life-sustaining machines and drugs that sometimes do little or nothing to alter the outcome.]

The philosophy underlying the program emphasizes palliative care for the terminally ill patient/family within a home care setting. Palliative care is described as total care in that attention is directed to the physical, emotional, and spiritual needs of the terminally ill patient, care is provided in an appropriate home environment supported by auxiliary services and programs, and supportive understanding of the needs of the family is provided during both the treatment and the bereavement processes.

[Improving the quality of life and maintaining the dignity of the individual are of major importance in a palliative care program.] In an effort to achieve these ends, attention is directed towards:

- treatment of the individual rather than the disease

- control and/or prevention of pain

- open communication between patient, staff, and family to assure the patient an opportunity to participate in making decisions regarding the treatment plan

- efforts to reduce the feeling of isolation by allowing the terminally ill to spend as much time as possible in the home.

In order to provide as much specialized care as possible within a home environment, to better serve the needs of terminally ill patients, and to maintain continuity of care, the traditional home health agency initiates a specialized palliative care program to care for these patients. The hospice program is designed in such a manner that the home environment serves as the coordinating unit for the total care of the terminally ill. The hospice program is an expansion and intensification of the types of care which are currently provided by the home health services.

The written goals and objectives of the hospice home care program are:

1. To control symptoms and pain which cause physical discomfort for the terminally ill through the use of clinical pharmacology and other supportive treatment modalities.

2. To arrange inpatient care as necessary which will

- evaluate the needs of the terminally ill,

- design a coordinated treatment plan for each individual,

- relieve discomfort when the individual is unable to cope with the debilitating effects of a terminal illness,

- provide relief for the family in caring for the terminally ill individual.

3. To provide home health care by trained professionals, paraprofessionals, and volunteers to approximately 100 patients per year.

4. To increase the amount of time which the terminally ill individual may spend in his own home.

5. To provide or arrange a supportive milieu consisting of chaplain service, interpersonal communication, and good medical treatment which will attempt to meet the emotional, spiritual, and psychological needs of the patient as well as the family.

6. To design and implement educational programs to increase awareness of the hospice care concept as well as the specific needs of the terminally ill patients and their families. Educational programs will be conducted for

- local medical community members,

- the general public,

- patients enrolled in the program,

- families of patients,

- palliative care program staff members and consultants,

- volunteers to the palliative care program.

7. To develop community based and/or alternative funding sources to insure the continuation of the palliative care program.

Most patients are referred to the program either by their attending physician or by service agencies within the area. According to hospice home care policy, the traditional home care clinical supervisor and the hospice nurse are responsible for making day-to-day admissions to the hospice program following the referral of the primary care physician. The hospice committee and other members of the hospice staff may be consulted when problems arise as well as for periodic review of admission criteria. Following admission to the program, a treatment plan is designed for the individual by the hospice staff under the direction of the patient's physician. Treatment is provided in the home by personnel supposedly trained to be sensitive to the emotional, physical, and psychological needs of the terminally ill patient. Through regular contact with the patients and their families, the agency seeks to monitor both patient and family needs and suggests additional medical, emotional, and spiritual services which may aid the patient and family to cope with the problems associated with a terminal illness.

The written criteria that define the population to be served by the hospice home care program in addition to normal admission standards of the home care agency are:

- diagnosis of malignant disease

- a disease state where the only appropriate therapy is palliative care and life expectancy is in terms of weeks or months rather than years

- consent authorization by the patient's primary physician

- presence of a primary care person who will assume responsibility for the patient care at home on a twenty-four hour basis

- the patient/family must be motivated and willing to enter the program.

Admission to the hospice may be denied for the following reasons:

- The individual lives outside of the delivery area.

- A primary care person is not available on a twenty-four hour basis.

- The patient does not have an attending physician who will assume responsibility for monitoring and supervising care provided to the patient by the hospice staff.

- Hospice care is inappropriate; a diagnosis of end stage disease has not been made.

In instances when the patient is not admitted to the hospice program, the staff will advise the patient's attending physician and/or the team regarding treatment modalities which best meet the needs of the individual.

A hospice interim protocol is designed to insure that hospice patients admitted to the acute or extended care facility will receive continuous care from members of the hospice team during their stay in the acute or extended care facility with periodic visits by the nurses, homemaker/home health aides, the social worker, and the volunteers of the hospice during the patient's hospitalization. The purpose of these visits is to

- assure the patient's family that the hospice team members are concerned about the patient and are interested in the patient's health.

- provide continuity in the overall treatment plans established by the patient's physicians.

- reassure the patient and family that the hospice staff looks forward to the patient's return to the home treatment program.

- ease the transition from the acute or extended care facility to the home.

- assist the hospital staff in understanding the special needs of the hospice patients.

[Readmission to the home care program is to occur after the patient's specific physiological problems have been treated in the acute or extended care facility and when the patient may be maintained in the home.] Since families of patients being readmitted to the home care program are often apprehensive about the patient's return, as well as about their ability to care for their relative, the hospice nurses seek to meet with both the patient and the family in the acute or extended care facility prior to the patient's return to the home in an effort to facilitate the transition.

One agency statistics from this model show a large hospice caseload from implementation--over 50 patients--with 26 percent still living at the end of the 8 1/2 month period. Of the deceased patients, 13 families were discharged and 26 are continued for bereavement counseling. The diagnoses of the patients are highest in cancer of the lung, metastatic adenocarcinoma, and breast cancer, with 74 percent over age 60 and 25 percent between 41 and 60 (1% under age 40). Fifty percent of the deaths occurred in the hospital, 40 percent died at home, and

10 percent in the nursing home. The average length of stay in the hospice program was between 1 - 2 months.

An evaluation procedure for the home care model hospice program measures the amount of change it has produced in the delivery of health care to the terminally ill. Indirect measurements developed through the use of several questionnaires are administered at periodic intervals. This program evaluation plan required for certified home health agencies provides a quality assurance mechanism which assesses the extent to which the agency's program is appropriate, adequate, effective, and efficient.

Staffing Patterns

Staff within the traditional home care agency include an executive director, administrative/supervisory staff, office staff, registered professional nurses, homemaker/home health aides, chore service workers, and social service staff serving approximately 450 active patients. Independent contractors may include a nutritionist, physical therapist, occupational therapist, and speech therapist. There is no clergy, psychologist, or psychiatrist on the traditional staff. Therefore, hospice patients are referred to their own clergy. Typically, administration of the hospice program is carried out by the home care executive director.

Initially a nurse is hired and trained to coordinate a hospice team; her title is nurse specialist in terminal illness. The nurse specialist in terminal illness is described as a registered professional nurse who has received specialized instruction and training in the physical, emotional, and spiritual care of patients with terminal illness. The nurse specialist provides direct care to patients requiring such services, and is responsible for assessment, planning, implementation, and evaluation of services; the nurse also serves as a consultant to other agency employees serving patients with terminal illness. The nurse specialist is directly responsible to the traditional home care clinical supervisor. This registered professional nurse specialist coordinates hospice services in the community making weekly rounds in the community hospital with the oncologists, and stopping at the social service department for referral coordination. Primary responsibility for the management of the bereavement program is assigned to the nurse specialist. The primary concern of the bereavement program is to assist the bereaved to cope with the crisis of death and the related adjustments associated with the loss of a relative.

In the home care model described all staff are trained in hospice care; however, selected registered professional nurses are used for hospice care for closer continuity and supervision. Other staff such as home health aides and social workers see both types of patients.

Resources Available

Volunteers and paid staff members complement one another in a firm team effort within the flexible framework of the agency. Trained volunteers provide family support, respite care, grocery shopping, and bereavement counseling under the supervision of the nurse specialist in terminal areas. Volunteer training consists of four sessions each of four hours duration covering hospice, the gift of self--caregivers must know themselves so they can be free to concentrate on the needs of patients and families--grief management, personal death awareness, exploration of feelings about disease and dying, loss and bereavement counseling, communication skills, and ceremonial rites. Grants frequently fund a director of volunteers position in order to extend the volunteer program. Hospice volunteers play an active role in the bereavement program providing supportive services to family members throughout their mourning and bereavement period following the death of the patient.

The community agencies that work closely with the home care hospice are Cancer Society, Area Agency on Aging, Department of Public Welfare, Child Welfare, and Mental Health/Mental Retardation. The hospice steering committee, comprised of the home health agency board representatives, assist the integration of hospice into the overall program to facilitate its implementation.

Funding Sources

As a certified traditional home health agency, costs of hospice home care skilled services are covered through the existing third-party reimbursement mechanism. Funding for hospice programs is sought from numerous sources (church, memorials, fraternities) and with minimal financial support. While the traditional home health service has always provided care to terminally ill patients, the restrictions of existing funding resources necessitated limitations in the type and duration of service provided. These limitations generally resulted in the need for institutionalization of the dying patient who requires twenty-four hour care, drug therapy, intravenous feedings, X-rays, or certain other laboratory services. Hospice patients, however, are visited as needed by the hospice care team at any time of the day or night and for any length of time.

ADVANTAGES AND DISADVANTAGES

Expansion into a new hospice program is good public relations for the traditional home care organization and, therefore, increases community support.

The traditional home care agency does provide the basic services and a firm foundation upon which hospice services can be built. With the background, experiences, and knowledge of home care services, an administrator with sensitivity, commitment and vision can develop a quality hospice program. Unfortunately, the hospice home care model tied in with a traditional visiting nurse association (VNA) has limitations and demonstrates more disadvantages than advantages.

The traditional VNA does have a sound organized training program for orientation and a formalized written evaluation program; both are required for certification as a home health agency and are critical to quality of care. Unlike other models, a formal educational program component for ongoing education to hospice staff, patient/family, and community is lacking. Limited administrative time and funding make it difficult for the development of an educational program since time constraints and funds dictate focus on patient services.

The traditional home care-based model has not formally coordinated inpatient and home care. They have limited defined linkages or arrangements for service with one or more service agencies or programs along the continuum of care between acute inpatient and home care services written into hospice program policies. In the home care model, the executive director responsible for other home care programs has limited time to spend for hospice administration unlike the other models with full-time administration. One can only speculate what effects this will have on the future of home care models. Attention to spiritual concerns, plans for funeral services, estate planning, and bereavement services have not been traditionally included in home health agency services, whereas these needs become the focus in a hospice program of care.

Administrative commitment to inclusion of a member of the clergy on the hospice care team to coordinate or directly provide spiritual counseling appears to reflect on the history of the development of each hospice program. The traditional home care model has not included a pastoral counselor as a member of the staff. Consequently, pastoral care services are lacking in the home care model.

The scope of the hospice care team in the traditional home care model was not as broad as in the other models of care. Approximately 25 percent of the hospice patients in the home health agency received services from an interdisciplinary team. Lack of funding may be a reason for limited expansion of the interdisciplinary team. This also may be due to lack of personnel and/or limited access to specialists and consultants. The informal community ties by the home health care model does not assure availability.

The physical therapist was rarely used, the psychiatrist was not used, and the social worker was involved in only 23 percent of the patients.

The survey conducted by the author showed that the number of volunteers in the home care model is limited compared to other models. This author feels that the traditional home care model described here does not utilize volunteers in the home care setting for a number of reasons, yet volunteers are an integral part of the hospice care team. Home base is not as visible to the public which limits volunteer involvement. Volunteers in home care work separately in individual homes and with individual patients which is not conducive to a central meeting place where many times volunteers like to work as a group. Consequently, the volunteer may receive less satisfaction from his or her assignments. Minimal use of the interdisciplinary team and lack of a formal ongoing educational program contribute to limited use of the volunteer. Due to limited training, staff are not skilled in comprehensive patient/family assessment which is necessary for assignment of the volunteer as a team component.

Pain and symptom control are considered extremely important in the care of hospice patients for all models underscoring the philosophy that if pain and symptoms are not under reasonable control, other comfort and caring measures are usually fruitless and may even be counterproductive. A person's pain threshold will vary according to mood and morale, and intensity of pain likewise. In the home care model, pain medication administered on a PRN (whenever necessary) basis more than around the clock is expected since family education is difficult, yet crucial in assessment of pain. Rossman (1979) comments that of 1500 British hospice patients, 70 percent arrived at the hospice, an inpatient facility, in severe pain. A British physician concluded that at least a fifth of dying hospice patients are in severe pain which could be relieved. The varied approaches to pain control found in the home care model appeared to be a problem because of the number of different primary physicians providing medical orders. Minimum use of pain control around the clock relates to not practicing antitumor therapy, a medical practice phenomenon.

Lack of coordination and continuity in home care is evidenced by the following discharge policies which are used only in the home care model. Discharge from the home care hospice occurs in one of the following ways in addition to normal standards for discharge:

> When the patient can no longer be successfully maintained in the home due to specific physiological problems which requires more intensive treatment that can be provided in a home. In such instances, the patient will be admitted to the acute or extended care facility for continued care and supervision by the appropriate physicians. In this instance, the Interim Protocol will be followed.

> When the patient died in the home care setting. In such instances, members of the hospice staff are available to

> - provide emotional support to family members.
>
> - assist in the transfer of the body to the funeral home if necessary.
>
> - notify the team of the patient's death.
>
> - assist the family in making any last minute funeral arrangements as needed.

These discharge policies then limit bereavement counseling services.

The home care hospice program has the distinct advantage of allowing their patients to remain in their own home with an appropriate support system under their control. A nurse specialist in hospice care provides the expertise necessary to plan, implement, and monitor the program. On the other hand, the lack of a medical director to provide specialist skills tends to limit medical direction based on hospice concepts and philosophy; for example, pain control as found in the medical record audit where only 23 percent of those patients with pain received pain medication around the clock.

As a certified home health agency, the existing reimbursement system covers home services like the community-based models. The disadvantages of the home care model are the failure to coordinate community resources, a lack of continuity of care, and a failure to use an interdisciplinary team as evidenced in medical record audit results where 5 percent of the patients received volunteer services and none received pastoral care. Lack of an institutional setting as part of the hospice program limits their services to hospice patients in the home. The home setting is not appropriate for everyone at all times, especially those who do not have a primary care person to provide care between home care visits.

Another disadvantage is the fact that the administrator of the hospice program is also responsible for other complex programs within the total home care organization. This limits the amount of time spent on hospice administration.

While the benefits of home care make it superior to other available options for both patient and family, it is a difficult commitment to make; it requires deliberation, thought, and careful planning. Home care is not a panacea effective for everyone just as hospice is not appropriate for everyone. The choice must be made by the entire caregiving group; especially the patient must participate in the decision.

Since home care is a component of all models, the advantages and disadvantages are summarized as evidenced by this author:

Advantages:

- The cost is considerably less than that of institutional care and is reimbursable either in part or totally by some health insurance plans.

- The family and patient have the opportunity to fully experience the final days as a family together without any restrictions except those they wish to impose.

- The patient and family retain much more control over the situation, therefore reducing feelings of hopelessness and helplessness.

- Invasive life-prolonging (or death-prolonging) procedures are unavailable in the setting but can be obtained if needed. They are less likely to be inappropriately used in a crisis.

- Food and activity can be geared toward usual lifestyle or preference.

- Hospice staff can help teach a family how to care for the ill person, monitor progress, and be available for problems and questions.

- Hospice staff, entering into the family system, has the opportunity to effect positive change in the patterns of communication and guide the family toward resolution of conflict.

Disadvantages:

- Families often do not understand how demanding the twenty-four hour care of a person can be; they can become exhausted yet refuse to accept help.

- Reimbursement of cost is often to some extent uncertain with unskilled care.

- Families may feel abandoned by the health care system and improperly prepared for the task of home care. Emergencies can trigger overwhelming anxiety.

- Unless the care is planned, the bulk of nursing responsibilities may fall upon the shoulders of one person, who becomes drained (Roche, 1980).

Hospice home care services vary among hospice models and are different than traditional home care. Differences in hospice home care and traditional home care are frequently discussed among traditional caregivers and hospice caregivers. Several problems are identified in the present system of care which are worthy of mentioning here since these problems clarify that traditional home care agencies often do not provide hospice care, even though many agencies claim they do.

First, the traditional home care agency does not provide services on a twenty-four hour coverage basis. Hospice patients and families may need several hours of support during the night and on weekends. More time is required in the homes of hospice patients. Families and patients as a unit of care need extended visits. Traditional agencies with limited volunteer services cannot relieve families to go shopping or have periods of time away from care of the patients.

Home care staff are also not presently trained in specialized terminal care, the grief process, how to give support, technical aspects of preparation of the body both physically and spiritually, preparation for funeral and ceremonial rites, and bereavement services. Hospice caregivers are given extensive education and training in all these specialized areas. Staff support programs do not exist in traditional home care agencies to allow staff to express their own grief after the death of a patient whom they become very close to while providing care.

And, most importantly, the traditional agency has limited reimbursement for unskilled care, extended visits, and bereavement visits.

Traditional hospitalization is extremely costly, with use of new technologies, the intensive care unit, and emergency medical mechanisms. In the hospital, the family cannot participate in patient care even though family members may have a very strong need to continue caring for that person they have cared for during their entire life. Within hospice programs the family has the opportunity to share the final days of life and participate in their care.

A difference is evident in home services provided through contract and those given directly by the hospice organization. The major differences occur in the length of time of the visit, type of team members visiting, whether visits are made jointly or by an individual, comprehensiveness of care, coordination of care, and degree of death and dying and bereavement counseling. Hospice care is supposed to be provided anytime within a twenty-four hour period for any length of time by various members of the team on the basis of need either individually or jointly. Hospice team members are supposed to become deeply involved with patients and their families providing an in-depth service and support including death, dying and bereavement counseling. Hospice team members are supposed to utilize existing resources as evidenced by the number of contacts and referrals on the medical record. Also the hospice team is each a member of a committee according to minutes and documentation of meetings. The team members meet frequently--daily on an informal basis as noted in the medical record and formally once weekly for an all-day session--to discuss and coordinate patient care unlike the brief coordination in traditional agencies.

In general, home care serves the patient's medical, social, economic, and spiritual interests by extending health care to their residence. In addition to providing continuity of care, the home health program shortens the length of hospital stay and, in some instances, obviates the need for hospitalization. This, in turn, promotes appropriate utilization of beds and other hospital facilities and reduces health care costs as evidenced in the discussion on home care costs. Home care provides the opportunity to continue or to modify patient teaching begun in the hospital. Factors in the home which may interfere with top quality patient care can be identified early and corrected. The hospice experiences by this author verify the important role of home care in terminal disease.

However, we must again emphasize that the home care model alone under the administration of a traditional home care agency, that is, a visiting nurse association, has limited team resources and lack of formal ties within the community. The absence of the interdisciplinary hospice team, according to hospice standards, indicates very limited expansion of the traditional program. It appears that use of the traditional cancer nursing team with nurses specially trained in oncology are being labeled hospice. This team perhaps has been expanded mainly in the area of bereavement. Also programs that can provide home care may have only little influence on care once institutionalization is necessary.

In their Ohio study, Brooks and Smyth-Staruch (1983) clarified the cost-effectiveness of hospice care by a comparison of the use of hospital and home care services among hospice study subjects with that of cancer decedents who also received home care services, but not within the framework of a hospice palliative care program. Hospice cancer decedents use substantially fewer days of hospital inpatient care and substantially more home care visits than the nonhospice cancer decedents on home care (Brooks and Smyth-Staruch, 1983). Hospice cost savings were realized by substituting less expensive home care visits for more expensive hospital days. Pryga and Bachofer (1983), writing on cost of care for the terminally ill, make it clear that demonstration of cost savings is one of the most difficult aspects of the current national debate. Comparison of the cost of caring for the terminally ill in both hospice care and traditional care is difficult due to inconsistent scope of services, variable use of volunteers, and effect of medical condition and family or primary care person services. Hospices are not currently required to provide all of the services in a comprehensive package. The extent to which volunteers provide direct patient care services can affect the hospice's costs, depending on whether the services would otherwise have been provided by paid hospice staff (e.g., homemaker services versus friendly visits). Also the capability and capacity of family/primary carepersons and the hospice patient's medical condition will result in varying degrees of success in substituting home care for inpatient care.

Reflecting on current hospice Medicare certification conditions of participation, the home care model as described in this chapter would not be eligible at this time for Medicare certification because of the required scope of services including both inpatient and home care and the professional management responsibility requirements. The question remains for the home care model administrator: Do we need to apply for hospice Medicare certification?

In his writing on home health care, Spiegel (1983) focuses on birth and death at home--generic issues in home care. His summary of the advantages and disadvantages of hospice home care and his evaluation of a home-based hospice serves as a reference in that the home care component of hospice appears to be favorable. If the VNA in a community has the financial or philanthropic/volunteer resources to provide those hospice services not covered by third-party payors and adequate capacity to deliver both inpatient and home care, perhaps other criteria discussed for quality of care could be met through careful planning and changes within the traditional system. Otherwise, another model of care should be explored as an alternative.

Home care may not always be feasible for two main reasons: (1) inadequate support systems, and (2) need for care is beyond the scope of expertise of willing family members.

QUALITY AND THE HOME CARE MODEL

The criteria necessary to assure quality care discussed in Part I of this book involve both direct and indirect patient care. The home care model described meets direct patient care by providing availability of twenty-four hour services to hospice patients, coordinating the patient/family as a unit of care, and offering a palliative care program. Indirectly, flexibility and continuity are incorporated into hospice care, traditional reimbursement for home care is an ongoing funding source, and an evaluation process is a component of a quality assurance program. However, criteria not met which involve direct patient care and limit quality hospice services are lack of pastoral care services, underutilization of volunteers, and lack of an expanded use of the IDG team. Bereavement services are not provided to all the families. As noted previously, the home care model does not have a formal ongoing staff and community educational program. Policies and procedures do not include symptom management and, as discussed earlier in this chapter, pain control is inconsistent among patients. Admission policies do not promote antitumor therapy for palliative purposes and use of diagnostic tests and treatments for symptom relief. Without separate administration and full-time management, hospice program progress can be impeded.

ADMINISTRATIVE CONSIDERATIONS

If a traditional home care model is selected, the quality concerns are important. The criteria not met would need to be studied thoughtfully to set up a hospice program. The hospice administrator must then address the barriers to quality services and seek mechanisms to overcome them.

The hospital-based home care program with central autonomous hospice administration is perhaps the ideal system of hospice care because of its flexibility and continuity. This conclusion is based on a significant finding of the author's research--the home care model alone is the least effective model in regard to quality of care. Both emotional and physical support can be provided whether the patient is in the hospital or at home. Even in the home setting the hospice care team has the resources of the hospital on which to rely if necessary. Since in philosophy the ideal model is a hospital-based home care program with an inpatient hospital unit--with central autonomous hospice administration which provides hospice care--patients can enter the program while hospitalized or enter the program while at home and can shift back and forth between settings as necessary. The inpatient hospital unit provides a setting where the professional staff are with the patients/families twenty-four hours a day, an advantage over scattered beds and home care. This allows the patient/family to feel more secure when death is imminent. Staff, patients, and families can feel that everything is being done for them. An atmosphere of relief enhances the quality of life. The hospital-based model research sites studied by the author did not have their *own* home care programs. They had to contract with existing agencies as discussed in Chapter 5 because of certificate of need laws in some states; this, in itself, limits control. Chapter 7 describes the freestanding model.

REFERENCES

Brooks, Charles H., and Kathleen Smyth-Staruch. (1983). *Cost Savings Of Hospice Home Care To Third-Party Insurers.* Cleveland, OH: Hospice

Council for Northern Ohio, Blue Cross of Northeast Ohio, and Case Western Reserve University.

Gold, Margaret. (1983). *Life Support: What Families Say About Hospital, Hospice and Home Care for the Fatally Ill.* Mount Vernon, NY: Consumers Union Foundation, Inc., Institute for Consumer Policy Research.

Pryga, Ellen A., and Henry J. Bachofer. (1983). *Hospice Care Under Medicare: A Working Paper.* Chicago: American Hospital Association, Office of Public Policy Analysis.

Roche, K.A. (1980). *Sharing the Experience of Death: A Manual of Family Care.*

Rossman, Parker. (1979). *Hospice.* New York: Fawcett Columbine.

Spiegel, Allen D. (1983). *Home Healthcare.* Owings Mills, MD: National Health Publishing.

Chapter 7

Freestanding Model

MODEL DESCRIPTION

A freestanding hospice facility is an independent hospice program which functions autonomously and not under the auspices of any other institution or agency. Arrangements for home care may be made with area home care organizations, or the hospice program could become a licensed/certified home health agency depending on the specific geographic area involved. Certificate of need regulations vary among states.

Community members become concerned when selecting a mechanism for inpatient services. In one instance during the formative stages when members of the community showed anxiety over the hospice program being hospital-based, two reasons became apparent: (1) that the hospital might become known as a "death" hospital; and (2) that money would be taken away from life support and given to terminal care. Nevertheless, acceptance of hospice as an appropriate way to respond to the health care vacuum that has existed for the dying patient can be seen by the number of new programs evolving, the media coverage, and the public and private financial support that is given to hospice programs at all levels. Costs of hospice care are much higher in the beginning when new services are started. Community support is necessary at all levels. Acceptance is a factor in the dilemma facing hospice today.

The amount of monies available and funding resources affect the varied models in terms of expansion and extent of services; however, they do not directly determine quality of services. The freestanding model requires unique planning in order to assure an ongoing funding resource through the existing reimbursement system as an acute or skilled facility or through specific state legislation such as in Connecticut.

Any freestanding hospice starting with grant monies have higher costs initially because those hospices tend to utilize paid staff rather than volunteers for nonreimbursable visits.

A TYPICAL FREESTANDING HOSPICE

Formal and Informal Structure

A freestanding hospice facility is an autonomous program with hospital and home care affiliations. Inpatient care supplements the home care program during times when the patient may temporarily need more intensive nursing care than can be provided at home or when the family needs a brief respite. The home care program utilizes the local visiting nurse association and, whenever possible, other community services. The home care capacity is sixty-five with an average caseload of fifty; an average of eight patients is usually in the inpatient component. The length of stay varies from one week to several months.

One program familiar to the author operated a sixteen-bed inpatient facility on a private estate that had been converted to accommodate hospice patients and their families. The concept of hospice care was brought to the local hospital by the president of the hospital's board of trustees, after a visit to St. Christopher's Hospice in London, England. He was greatly impressed by the warmth and support that hospice care provided the patients and was interested in establishing a program based on these principles but adapted to the specific needs of the community.

A task force composed of hospital board members along with both professional and lay community members was appointed to perform a feasibility study. Physicians, community leaders, prominent citizens, church, service, and professional groups, and educational institutions were approached to promote interest and support. Through the efforts of professional volunteers, the first group of volunteers which included nurses and lay individuals was trained.

With a nucleus of volunteers trained and ready to begin, the first patient was accepted into the program at which time an extensive home care program was begun on a twenty-hour-a-day, seven-days-a-week basis, as a special project under the auspices of the States Division of Alternative Health Systems. The hospice was granted certificate of need approval to operate as a hospice demonstration project in that state. The initial caseload was limited to five patients and their families due to limited funding and the commitment to provide excellence in services. As funding increased so did the census. Today an average hospice serves an average census of thirty patients and their family members.

Program Components

The freestanding model is a program of medical, spiritual, and social support services established to enable terminally ill cancer patients to die at home. The philosophy of the freestanding program managerially distinct from its parent organization is the provision of humane, compassionate, palliative medical and social care to cancer patients, and their families. The primary goals of hospice care are to provide the support necessary to help the patient die with dignity and to minimize the destructive impact of cancer death on the surviving family members. While the home care program receives primary emphasis, a small back-up inpatient facility of sixteen or less beds is also available for times when the patient cannot remain at home. In order to provide the highest quality of service, hospices frequently limit their caseload to thirty families.

Criteria for admission to a freestanding hospice program typically includes:

- Referral from the patient's primary care physician.

- A completed course of definitive treatment for cancer with a diagnosis of end stage disease.

- A prognosis in terms of weeks to months, as opposed to years.

- A primary care person, either a family member, a live-in friend, or paid companion, who must be able to attend the patient on an around-the-clock basis.

- Residence in one of the towns that lie within an approximately thirty minute driving radius of the facility.

A coordinating team comprised of the heads of the various disciplines of hospice meets weekly to review patients' conditions and the effectiveness of the treatment plans.

Admission to the inpatient unit occurs through the mutual planning of the patient, family, and hospice team and must be approved by the hospice coordinating team. The patient's physician must be in agreement with the plan, and the family must be available to participate actively in the patient's care while in the unit. The inpatient facility is largely used to provide respite for families and for pain and symptom control with the hope of the patient returning to the home. It may, in some situations, also be the appropriate choice for the patient's last few days of life.

A program to alleviate identified problems is worked out with the patients; the goal is to enable the patient and family to live as normally as possible during the duration of the illness. The hospice staff seek to assist in the contact with appropriate community agencies to utilize existing services for carrying out the plans of care whenever possible. When additional or more extensive support is needed, hospice provides this assistance directly based on written policies. Staff members meet with the patient and family on a regular basis to monitor program effectiveness and to make any adjustments necessary for changing situations.

After the death of the patient, hospice staff and volunteers continue to visit during bereavement, providing counseling, financial help, companionship, and when necessary, referral to community programs. This aspect is coordinated by a director of bereavement follow-up who may be a nurse or a medical social worker with certified counseling credentials. Bereavement interviews are conducted on a gradually decreasing basis for up to twelve months, a shorter period of time than some American hospices.

The secondary focus of the hospice program was that the freestanding inpatient facility intended to meet the specific needs of those cancer patients who for medical, psychological, or other reasons, need to be away from home for periods of time or to die. Efforts are, however, directed toward helping these patients remain in or return to their homes whenever possible. Through observation on the initial site visit of one hospice, the freestanding inpatient facility is run much as a home would be, which--according to interviews with professional staff nurses--fosters the development of a sense of community and mutual caring and support among all members of hospice. Interaction between staff, patients, and visitors through both informal and planned gatherings was observed. One patient was permitted solitude upon his request. According to written policy, there is no restriction to visiting. According to the director of nursing, the staff of the freestanding inpatient facility and of the home care program coordinate each patient's program to maintain a continuity of services although the role of community agencies is discontinued while the patient is in the inpatient unit.

Hoping to serve as a prototype for other institutions, one freestanding inpatient hospice has a comprehensive education and training component included as an integral part of this model. This component is funded through a grant from the National Institute of Mental Health and a regional Office of Consumer Health Education.

Ongoing in-service training programs as well as bimonthly "rap sessions" are held for hospice staff and volunteers. The "rap sessions" offer the chance to discuss both issues arising on specific cases and general problems or themes confronted in patient care, as well as the needed opportunity for staff and volunteers to meet together as a team, experience a sense of community, vent frustrations, and share successes. In-service training programs are designed to increase knowledge of medical, psychosocial, and recreational theories and advances, and to further the ongoing exploration and development of individual thoughts and feelings. The staff psychologist, chaplain, and volunteer director are also available on an individual basis should specific needs arise.

A patient's day in the freestanding facility as observed by the author while interviewing staff nurses appeared to involve very close supervision and constant supportive care by registered professional nurses. Two patients were seen sitting comfortably in the large, beautifully decorated living room; two professional nurses sat with them and conversed about daily events--football, nice weather, and current events. A patient weeping brought special attention from one professional nurse who discussed the frequency of such emotional episodes. Various patients hugged and held the hand of the professional nurse. A family member was present with one patient playing cards at a round table within the same living room. A snack and milkshakes were brought to the patients in the middle of the afternoon with encouragement from the nurses regarding the importance of their nutrition. The facility had a spacious yard with a pond nearby. A nurse was seen wheeling a patient to the pond as they both sat in the sun and conversed pointing to the trees, birds, and ducks watching the beauty and activities of nature. The two patients ate their meals at a round table in the living room with the nurses.

A television program relating patient activities in this facility showed mingling of patients, families, and volunteers during group activities with both inpatients and home patients. A nurse stated during the site visit that occasionally a home patient will spend the day at the freestanding facility because he/she cannot stay alone and the primary care person either works or needs respite. Two inpatients were present during this visit with three registered professional nurse members of the hospice team in attendance.

Staffing Patterns

The hospice team in a freestanding facility typically includes physician, registered and licensed practical nurses, a social worker, clergy, a psychologist, and volunteers working to coordinate and complement already existing community nursing and counseling services.

Twenty-four hour on-call services are also provided to hospice patients and families at home in crisis. The freestanding inpatient nurse staff receives the requests for help and, if needed, can dispense a home care nurse on an "immediate response" basis.

Resources Available

Over 200 trained volunteers may assist a hospice team. The training sessions consist of twenty hours of lecture with six hours of practicum at a nursing home in the beginning and then at the freestanding facility. Through a training grant, a volunteer training manual can be published by a hospice. A brochure for caregivers states that volunteers are an essential part of a hospice care program and are utilized as extensions of the patient's family to assist them in helping themselves. They are also utilized as extensions of the professional components of the hospice team and help ensure that this aspect of care remains both effective and appropriate in meeting patient/family needs and desires. Personal services by volunteers for primary care person relief consist of friendly visits, in-home recreation, transportation, assistance, reading to patient, letter writing, child care, and light housekeeping.

Volunteer training programs are planned to provide a background of information that will help in understanding the dying patient and his family. It is also intended to direct the volunteer's attention to his or her own feelings and attitudes toward death and loss. Each weekly session, therefore, encompasses not only factual material relevant to the hospice concept but also opportunities for each volunteer to look at his or her emotional reactions to death as he may have met it in the past and what he may expect in the future in his role as a volunteer working with the terminally ill.

Community services that typically work in association with the hospice home care program include the County Visiting Nurse Association, the County Homemakers, American Cancer Society, and Family Services. The large corps of specially screened and trained volunteers provide additional homemaking and housekeeping aid, transportation, socialization, companionship, and other support services.

Funding Sources

The National Cancer Institute (NCI) provided funding for a limited number of hospice programs. One program was funded for a three-year period after which unavailable ongoing funding brought about a reorganization which resulted in an inpatient hospital-based unit with a reduction of beds by two-thirds. During the time of the NCI contract there were no direct charges for services provided by the hospice. However, the average daily cost to hospice for the provision of the total care plan has been fifty dollars per day per patient. Patients and relatives are requested to consider making a contribution to the hospice in accordance with their means. Simultaneously, hospices continue to explore additional means of funding from grants and foundations, from corporations and organizations (both secular and religious), from the community at large (both professional and lay), from all who support the hospice concept and this program--and who may someday have need of services.

Seawing Hospice* was formally a freestanding hospice model of care funded for a three-year period through a contract with the National Cancer Institute which ended in September, 1980. During the three-year period Seawing Hospice, affiliated with Seawing Hospital, operated a sixteen-bed inpatient facility on a private estate that had been converted to accommodate hospice patients and their families. Inpatient care in the Seawing Hospice supplemented the Seawing home care program during times when the patient may temporarily need more intensive nursing care than can be provided at home or when the family needs a brief respite. Despite many months of long-range planning, the original freestanding unit had to close due to lack of funding. It moved to Seawing Hospital in February 1981, offering a small five-bed inpatient unit; it continued the home care program through contract with the local Visiting Nurse Association (VNA). This type of affiliation allows for third-party reimbursement, continuity of patient care, and utilization of other services the VNA offers to their patients, such as physical and speech therapies.

---

* "Seawing Hospice" is a pseudonym for one of the hospices utilized as a research site by the author.

ADVANTAGES AND DISADVANTAGES

Unlike the other models, an autonomous administration with concentration on hospice patients alone within a unique facility provides a homelike environment conducive to the dying patient and his/her family. The resourceful administration and interdisciplinary team is a valuable combination and an advantage in administering hospice services. A freestanding facility has the advantage of sufficient flexibility in implementation of policies to make hospice care workable.

The major disadvantage may be lack of on-going funding. Economically, the freestanding model is difficult to maintain without on-going grant monies and third-party reimbursement mechanisms. The New Haven Connecticut Hospice is a unique example where licensure was obtained through new regulations in the state of Connecticut under the section in the public health code on short-term special hospital care and regulations for on-going reimbursement. A separate hospice with its own board gives priority to the terminally ill. This organizational structure is therefore recommended since the hospice would then have an administration with a different basic commitment. A separate facility or at least a separate unit is needed to give leverage and flexibility to the demonstration of hospice methods and is recommended as a base to change the health care system.

To summarize, therefore, the advantages of a freestanding facility are the autonomous administration, an administrative team representing various disciplines, a commitment to a program of care by a specialized interdisciplinary care team who focus on expert palliative care, unlimited resources within the overall institution setting, and the facilitation of coordination of care within the community. The major disadvantage, if not authorized as a traditional or special hospital facility, is inability to bill third-party payment sources for services provided.

The Government Accounting Office review of hospice activity in the United States indicated that freestanding hospice costs are substantially higher than those associated with home care and community-based programs. (U.S. General Accounting Office, 1979).

Some areas of the country simply have a population which is too small to sustain a separate facility. Such areas, therefore, are forced to apply the hospice concept within a hospital or nursing home setting.

Another advantage of a freestanding hospice facility is that in a separate facility a family physician interested in continuing to visit the patient can do so without feeling the pressures of existing procedures and negative attitudes within the hospital which he regularly visits.

It is argued that the hospital provides more resources for the hospice team to draw upon than a separate facility. However, the terminally ill patient does not need to pay a share for all the unneeded services and equipment which traditionally represents curative treatment; the existence of such services often results in a resident physician applying "heroic measures" to hospice patients (Rossman, 1979).

It is further argued that the degree of sensitive, loving, and compassionate caregiving needed cannot always be provided in a hospital where habitual practices make change difficult. The complexity of hospital administration alone with its priorities of finances and space creates limitations that can be overcome by a freestanding hospice facility.

QUALITY AND THE FREESTANDING MODEL

The goal of the freestanding model is to establish a program that will improve the quality of care for the terminally ill cancer patient, while paying strict attention to performance standards and patient data to help establish the cost-effectiveness of the program. This continuing assessment is carried out through feedback of patients and staff, the maintenance and review of extensive problem-oriented records, and the accumulation of detailed cost-of-services data. The administrator expects that the overall cost of hospice care in the future will be lower than the cost of that being rendered at present.

Direct care criteria met by the freestanding model were provision of twenty-four hour service, use of the interdisciplinary team, treating the patient/family as a unit of care, provision of palliative care, and continuity of care.

Indirect care criteria met were central administration and coordination of services, program flexibility, and a formalized commitment to an educational program and an evaluation program.

Direct care criteria not met from the author's survey were pastoral care provided for only 17 percent of patients studied, volunteer services provided for only 48 percent of patients studied, bereavement services provided for only 75 percent of patients/families studied, and pain control provided for only 72 percent of patients studied. The limited pastoral care services and volunteer services may relate to their staffing and funding. A relationship may exist between increase in use of the pain control criterion and 100 percent use of the interdisciplinary team to handle the multi-dimensional needs of patients. The freestanding facility does not include active antitumor therapy or diagnostic studies as components of their care.

ADMINISTRATIVE CONSIDERATIONS

As discussed earlier, the lack of a reimbursement mechanism within a freestanding facility provides a major administrative concern. Hospice planners must look at grant or foundation monies as only start-up costs for specific aspects of a program with a mechanism for on-going reimbursement built into the initial program design. This assures continuity and provides a positive focus for on-going quality services. At the same time, select administrators/supervisors can be recruited and chosen with adequate planning to accomplish the long-range goals for a viable program. Without plans for funding sources, a freestanding unit inevitably faces a major barrier to a successful program of care.

The tremendous growth potential is staggering; however, the key to developing a freestanding hospice program model is sound financial planning, market research, and risk analysis and structuring alternatives through strategic planning.

One 300-bed hospital in Texas is constructing a freestanding twenty-bed hospice facility to serve a twenty-six-county area. Hospice of Northern Virginia is accredited by Joint Commission on Accreditation of Hospitals as both a hospice and a hospital. In addition to the accreditation, Hospice of Northern Virginia is also certified by Medicare as a hospice, home health agency, and a hospital. These are prime examples of the need and growth potential of hospice (NHO, 1984).

Into this breach between home care that is too often impractical and hospital care that is too often inadequate may move the institutional hospice. Designed to combine the skills of the one with the warmth and welcome of the other, the hospice approach is built upon a profound understanding of the interweaving of the psychological and physical strands. It differs from the hospital, which is set up to serve different clienteles with different needs, fears, and desires; the hospice aims to preserve the patient's dignity and autonomy in the face of the most terrible of truths. A number of techniques are utilized, including the building of strong health teams who have positive self-regard as well as respect for their duties and their patients. Hospice sets out to eliminate regulations that inconvenience patients to no worthwile end. A feeling of community among patients and between patients, staff, and families is created through family participation in treatment, continuing and sympathetic psychiatric assistance, and other means. Thus, though dying is necessarily a private matter, corrosive and embittering loneliness is minimized and the web of interpersonal support strengthened. While contact is maintained with the outside world and the patient's loved ones, efforts are made to help the patient accept death with a measure of hope; hospice respects the patient's humanity in dozens of minor ways that can, in sum, make a major difference. All of this is informed by the recognition that the depression, worry, and anxiety that accompany terminal illness are often more debilitating than the ailment itself (Craven and Wald, 1975).

Freestanding hospice institutions have been the goal of many fledgling hospice programs--a goal that unfortunately is not practical in today's economy and in today's system. The cost of establishing the facility is prohibitive, and the system already contains more efficient alternatives.

REFERENCES

Craven, Joan, and Florence S. Wald. (1975). Hospice Care for Dying Patients. *American Journal of Nursing* 75:1819.

National Hospice Organization. (1984). *Hospice News* 2(7):6.

Rossman, Parker. (1979). *Hospice.* New York: Fawcett Columbine.

U.S. General Accounting Office. (1979). *Hospice Care--A Growing Concept in the United States.* HRD 79-50, March 6.

Chapter 8

Community-Based Model

MODEL DESCRIPTION

The community-based model, in many ways, is perhaps the purest form of hospice. The community-based program provides hospice services directly and coordinates existing services, a model which does not have to fit into an existing organizational structure.

Some authors when discussing the community-based hospice describe an all-volunteer program that depends on fundraising for survival. However, this author refers to a community-based model as an independent hospice program which becomes a certified home care agency, seeks affiliations, and coordinates existing services. This approach reduces fragmentation, avoids duplication, and provides a setting for a continuum of care within a well-planned organizational structure with autonomy.

A community-based program has the unique feature of community participation in a program of care which, in fact, can become *their* program and *their* hospice with a deeper feeling of commitment and self-involvement.

A TYPICAL COMMUNITY-BASED HOSPICE

Formal and Informal Structure

Community-based hospices do vary as to organizational structure. However, program components become similar.

One community-based program studied by this author functioned under the auspices of a parent organization which was a religiously-affiliated welfare service.

Early in 1979, the parent organization of this program received notification of a large grant of approximately $180,000 from Health, Education and Welfare, Administration on Aging for the development of a three-year demonstration program of care for the terminally ill elderly patient (fifty-five and over) to be called Lady Helena.* This community-based research site is one originally funded solely through monies for the aged.

The board of directors of the parent organization hired the director of Lady Helena and the nurse coordinator one month later. The director of hospice directs the overall program and provides staff leadership reporting to the parent organization executive director, hospice program advisory committee, and parent organization board of directors. The training and orientation of staff began immediately, with the assistance of consultants from the Connecticut Hospice and other agencies. Office space was secured from a local college located in the county seat and city most centrally located in that county. The offices were furnished and supportive personnel joined the hospice team.

According to the administrator, a twenty-member all-volunteer advisory committee for Lady Helena Hospice was appointed by the board of directors of the parent organization. The advisory committee meets monthly and acts in an advisory capacity to the board of directors and executive director of the parent organization, and to the director of Lady Helena Hospice. The advisory committee is divided into four subgroups: The program planning and evaluation subcommittee, public information subcommittee, legislative subcommittee, and the committee for funding and development.

A review of the history revealed that charting systems and nursing care policies were established, information forms and an information retrieval system were developed by a human services consultant association, and bereavement and follow-up care policies were determined.

Further review of the history brought forth the scope of this model in that the parent organization, the sponsoring agency, has been providing care for the ill and the elderly since 1958 when it was established as an independent corporation by representatives of congregations now belonging to a church synod in America. Presently the parent organization operates two facilities headquartered in the same geographic area, a community/regional program of human services, and the hospice care program employing more than 230 persons throughout the county. One facility is a community of care for the aging which provides both residential and skilled nursing care. At present, the home provides residential care to 108 residents in its domiciliary care program and skilled nursing care to sixty-one patients. The facility is constituted as a geriatric facility, with admissions intended for persons sixty-two years of age or older, and is certified by both Medicare and Medicaid programs for its skilled nursing patients.

The second facility, a 104-bed skilled nursing facility (SNF), through contract agreement provides inpatient care (four beds) for the patients participating in the Lady Helena Hospice Program. While it is constituted to serve persons over the age of sixteen in need of skilled nursing care, its census is

---

* Lady Helena is a pseudonym for one of the community-based hospices utilized as a research site by the author.

nearly always constituted by the ill elderly. According to the hospice director, Lady Helena Hospice staff visit hospice patients at regular intervals throughout the patient's stay at the skilled nursing facility and confer at regular intervals about hospice patients and the interrelationship of both parent services divisions. Lady Helena Hospice reimburses the skilled nursing facility its daily rate for services should third-party payment not be available. Lady Helena Hospice provides needed in-service training to the SNF staff.

Lady Helena Hospice, a coordinated home care and in-facility program, provides palliative and supportive services to patients/families suffering from a diagnosed terminal illness and having a limited life span during the terminal stages, after death, and during bereavement.

Lady Helena Hospice completed the certification process for becoming a home care agency after three years of service. Up to that time they utilized local Home Health Services, a traditional VNA agency, through a contract agreement to provide some of the home care services, specifically part-time public health nursing and home health aide. However, since coordination had been difficult, the Lady Helena director felt a need to provide all home care services.

In contrast, Hospice of Pa., Inc.,* an independent community-based model, was developed without a parent organization.

Hospice of Pa., Inc., a private voluntary nonprofit organization, coordinates a program of hospice care in an urban and rural community of approximately 250,000 people. Hospice of Pa., Inc. was established in May 1978 through a small grant from Elm Park Corporation, a local nonprofit group involved in housing for the elderly. The board of directors of Elm Park Corporation felt a deep commitment to the concept and philosophy of hospice care for the terminally ill and, therefore, formed this new corporation. Hospice of Pa., Inc. has a fifteen-member board of directors, an eighteen-member professional advisory committee headed by a local physician, and a twenty-member community advisory committee. Additional funds have been received through contributions, memorials, and fundraising efforts. In May 1978, through a pilot project with a local group of oncologists, Hospice of Pa., Inc. accepted its first patient. A member of this oncology group is one of the medical directors for hospice. In March 1980, Hospice of Pa., Inc. became a certified home health agency for Medicare and Medicaid and, at the same time, became an approved agency for Blue Cross reimbursement. Hospice of Pa., Inc. has been administered by this author, a registered professional nurse who holds a masters degree in public administration and a doctorate in public health.

In the summer of 1983, Hospice of Pa. Foundation was incorporated to act as a holding corporation for the subsidiary corporations. Through a matching grant from a local foundation, the Foundation was able to hire an individual as president and chief executive officer for hospice programs utilizing the original

---

* Hospice of Pa., Inc., is the program with which the author is affiliated. For purposes of the research a graduate student not affiliated with the organization collected the data.

administrator as a part-time management consultant. Currently the Foundation provides all management services to Hospice of Pa., Inc. The Foundation is actually engaged in the management of programs through contract and promotes continuing sensitive care service to the chronic and terminally ill. These services include in-home outpatient rehabilitative and planned inpatient rehabilitative programs that focus upon patient and family acceptance of the lifestyle changes brought on by a chronic condition. A Hospice Institute is planned for research and education which will provide funding sources for future program development. Hospice Foundation is the property owner with a major responsibility for fundraising. Hospice of Pa., Inc. currently provides all home care, outpatient, and other program services from a building owned by the Foundation.

As of November 1983 Hospice of Pa., Inc. received certification as a hospice for the new Hospice Benefit under the Medicare program and in October 1984 became a certified CORF* program to complete a continuum of care. Contracts are held with local hospitals and nursing homes for provision of inpatient services.

In addition, three inpatient units are being planned as demonstration projects with a total of thirty-five skilled nursing beds and six acute beds to be staffed and managed by Hospice of Pa., Inc. Such units will apply the hospice philosophy of care to those individuals and families with life-threatening conditions for short-term rehabilitative services.

Hospice of Pa., Inc. has planned a hospice care center for all services including sixty skilled beds--a project which momentarily requires additional funding to decrease the cost per bed--to be built on land donated by the Congregation of the Immaculate Heart of Mary at a future date.

Program Components

In Lady Helena, the community-based hospice, program components include home care, bereavement counseling, and education.

Written policy states that to be admitted to the hospice program the patient should

- be diagnosed as having a terminal illness with a limited prognosis.

- be a resident of the county.

- be receiving chemotherapy or radiotherapy for palliative purposes only.

- consent to these services.

- have the consent of the attending physician.

---

* Comprehensive Outpatient Rehabilitation Facility.

- preferably have a primary care person in the home.

Medical, nursing, social service, pastoral, and bereavement visits are coordinated with the continuous assessment of the patient and family needs at the weekly patient review conference. An on-going evaluation of the program is conducted by the program planning and evaluation subcommittee of the hospice advisory committee. Community physicians who have referred patients to the program are also involved in the evaluation of the care given to Lady Helena Hospice patients. According to the hospice director, the Lady Helena Hospice home care program has been very well received by the patient and families who have been involved and their enthusiasm has been regarded as most encouraging.

According to the director, Lady Helena Hospice is developing a learning/teaching center for the study of terminal illness and related issues. In-service training sessions have been held regularly; topics include symptom control in terminal illness, legislative relations, management of grief, temper control, leadership, and financing of a hospice program.

A review of statistics reveals that the program reached full capacity within six months with fifteen patients and families under care. Since that time, the patient census has varied. The staff recognizes the need for continued public information dissemination to increase the number of referrals. During the first year, 53 patients/families were served with 1,256 home visits, 89 bereavement visits, and 60 volunteers providing 1,017 hours of service. The following year, 83 patients/families were seen for 1,319 visits, 142 bereavement visits, and 1,577 hours of service from 90 volunteers. Within two-and-a-half years, Lady Helena Hospice had served 136 patients/families, most of whom have been elderly due to age restrictions placed on hospice by the Department of Health and Human Services/Administration on Aging. The daily patient census was 18 to 20 living patients/families, along with the continued responsibility of bereavement counseling to the 60 family members of deceased hospice patients.

The community-based model with two research sites is the only model which provides both coordinated inpatient care and direct home care, the reverse of the institutional models.

The components of another example of a community-based model, the Hospice of Pa., Inc. coordinated program include the following

- Coordinated inpatient hospice care in both hospitals and nursing homes
- Direct home health hospice care
- Education
- Volunteer services
- Bereavement counseling
- Outpatient services

According to written policy, Hospice of Pa., Inc. offers patients the opportunity to receive their services in a health care facility or at home. Following the agency philosophy--those faced with a life-threatening illness need more than traditional home care--the hospice team has been trained to provide the needed services in a health facility or in a patient's home.

The overall goals and objectives set forth by Hospice of Pa., Inc. board of directors are:

- To manage terminal disease in such a way that patients can live with their loved ones as they are dying, that their loved ones can go on living afterward with a minimum of problems, and that patients receive the best in medical and clinical interdisciplinary services available.

- To identify issues, questions, and problems related to the implementation of the hospice concept and to develop and evaluate solutions and innovative approaches that may advance the state of the art.

- To create dissemination and demonstration capacities that can lead to adaptation and replication of the practices of the proposed hospice program.

- To evaluate the effectiveness, efficiency, and impact of the hospice program in terms of patient/family services, cost/benefits, and potential multiplier effect.

Agency admission criteria now state that Hospice of Pa., Inc. accepts patients of any age faced with a life-threatening illness. Hospice of Pa., Inc. admission criteria are more expansive than all other research sites/models in that there is no limited prognosis and a patient can be on active curative chemotherapy or radiation therapy as well as blood and platelet therapy. Expansion of eligibility criteria resulted from a community need and demand-- based on a high elderly and chronic disease population requiring application of hospice care principles. A person may be referred to the program by a physician, nurse, a member of the family, a social worker, a clergyman, a friend, or by a neighbor. However, patients must be under the care of a physician who agrees that hospice referral is appropriate.

According to written policy, Hospice of Pa., Inc. coordinates and participates with other agencies as well as all hospitals and nursing homes in the community. Other agencies and programs include the Community Hospital Oncology Programs, American Cancer Society, Area Agency on Aging, Meals on Wheels, and Children's Bureau. Registered professional nurses and clinical social workers function as hospital coordinators who visit the hospitals on a regular basis to coordinate services and plan for discharge from hospital to home and home to hospital.

Based on admission policy, a clinical evaluation team--composed of physicians, a nurse-coordinator, and a medical social worker--evaluates patients seeking admission and is the authority in determining the eligibility and in designing and implementing a comprehensive plan of hospice care for the patient and his or her family. All patients/families reviewed receive a plan of care based on the professional findings of the hospice team to determine the degree of hospice involvement. Those patients/families who are accepted by the agency for treatment begin to receive specified services immediately. Services continue as prescribed for as long as needed by patient/family, including the hospice standard of bereavement counseling following the death of the patient. The clinical social worker initially does a psychosocial evaluation and then provides the psychosocial support services. Additional support offered by the hospice system differs according to the patient's required needs and may include the services of a speech therapist, physical therapist, occupational therapist, and services of a home health aide as well as other members of the interdisciplinary team.

Based on the history of Hospice of Pa., Inc., volunteers--both professional and nonprofessional--are an essential aspect of the hospice. According to the volunteer manual, these volunteers are screened by the nurse-coordinator upon completion of their formal training as to their proficiency and eligibility. Their training consists of six one-session seminars, each of which is two hours in duration, and is designed for those who wish to provide support and companionship to persons and families who are experiencing terminal illness. The training seminars for hospice volunteers are conducted by members of the clinical evaluation team and interdisciplinary team and are the shared responsibility of all staff members. Over 300 volunteers have been trained. Two volunteer coordinators are responsible for all components of volunteer services-- training, on-going education, coordination, and assignments.

Personnel employed by this agency vary their time input to allow for fluidity of service delivery in compliance with the hospice philosophy which renders round-the-clock service. According to agency policy, administrative and professional as well as clerical staff are required to attend the on-going supportive functions and educational sessions of the hospice program. These sessions relate to maintaining public relations, informative fiscal matters, operational procedures, and so on, as directed by the hospice board of directors and/or its committees.

Agency statistical reports show that the current active caseload of this agency consists of approximately 150 chronic and terminally ill patients with the additional families receiving bereavement counseling. According to agency minutes, the hospice board has extended the usual period of bereavement counseling from twelve months to an extended length of time--eighteen months or longer if required by the family or found necessary upon review by the team. In 1983, Hospice of Pa., Inc. served 469 patients/family with 12,681 house visits to patients and 426 bereavement visits to families. In addition, 712 volunteer visits and 669 senior companion visits were made. Senior companions provide respite-type services for four hours a day to hospice patients through a federally funded program for the elderly. Senior companions are coordinated through the volunteer program and are a valuable expansion of hospice services.

According to the bereavement statement, bereavement counseling by Hospice of Pa., Inc. is offered by a professional nurse who is a certified counselor, and by a continuing care team member (a trained volunteer for low-risk patients) assigned to the specific case. The nurse-counselor serves as coordinator of the bereavement program as discussed in Chapter 3.

Hospice of Pa., Inc. arranges weekly staff meetings which are conducted both informally and formally. The purpose of these meetings is to improve patient care as well as to keep each team member abreast of new developments in their own and related fields. Interdisciplinary team conferences are scheduled every Friday to review the plan of care for each patient and to revise as needed. Upon recommendations by the psychiatric consultant, these sessions are also designed to anticipate and forestall problems of stress affecting the staff adversely to prevent the possible loss of valuable trained staff members. The staff counselor plans additional staff support sessions on a regular basis which include all levels of staff; each level has separate sessions. The coordinator of the bereavement program also serves as the staff support person. The volunteer coordinator plans a monthly seminar which specifically includes hospice volunteers. In these instances, board members and staff actively participate or coordinate in planning the scheduled activities. Everyone associated with hospice is invited to attend these monthly seminars including family members of patients who wish to have clarified some phase of hospice not fully grasped by them. The son of a deceased patient acts as a patient/family representative in making presentations about hospice. To maintain community relations, hospice presentations or seminars are periodically held in hospitals at all levels as well as presented to service groups, for example, Parent Teachers Associations, News Club, Lions Organizations, Women's Clubs and so on to maintain public awareness of hospice services as evidenced in the community presentation manual.

Through planning by the community advisory committee, Hospice of Pa., Inc. has established its own transportation committee. An interested public-minded citizen who owns an ambulance currently provides this service when it is needed, regardless of the patient's ability to pay.

Based on agency policy, no terminally ill patient is ever rejected by Hospice of Pa., Inc. because of his or her inability to pay for services rendered. As of July 1, 1981, those eligible under Title XX, now the Adult Block Grant Program, are covered for bereavement counseling and homemaker services. Currently, the Hospice of Pa., Inc. executive committee is seeking additional funding resources through a contract for service with United Way for bereavement services.

Staffing Patterns

To further meet goals and objectives, Lady Helena Hospice--as documented in the background statement and agency purpose--offers to persons who are terminally ill an opportunity to live at home and to die at home, with their pain and other symptoms controlled, comforted and supported by family members and familiar surroundings. To make this possible, Lady Helena Hospice offers the following staff:

- A physician who is especially sensitive to the needs of the dying person and who is trained in the pharmacology of pain and symptom control.

- Specially trained registered nurses, who visit in the home on a regular or emergency basis depending on need.

- A social worker/counselor, who will counsel the patient and family regarding their psychological, social, and financial needs.

- A chaplain, who will assure that the patient's and family's needs for spiritual care are being met.

- A support system of volunteers with a variety of interests and skills, who will be matched to the needs of the patient and family as these needs are identified.

- An administrative support system provided by the Lady Helena Hospice office, and by the administrative facilities and personnel of the Welfare Service.

Visits to patient homes vary from daily to weekly by members of the hospice care team. The medical record included narrative notes by the nurse and social worker regarding an initial joint visit with subsequent visits made by the registered professional nurse, social worker, chaplain, and volunteers.

Hospice of Pa., Inc. staff presently consists of administrative and clerical personnel, nurses, social workers, physicians, physical therapist, occupational therapist, speech therapist, respiratory therapist, nutritionist, consulting psychiatrist and pharmacist, clergy, and home health aides who coordinate services with other agencies in human services. According to agency policy, members of the team assist the family in coping with the emotional and physical effects of the illness at home.

The staffing pattern of this agency includes physicians (an oncologist and a medical internist), nurse-coordinators, registered professional nurses, enterostomal therapist*, licensed practical nurses, medical social workers, social work assistants, home health aides, physical therapists, speech therapists,

---

* An enterostomal therapist is a registered nurse certified through special training to provide specialized skin care and "ostomy" care. She also becomes a consultant to other nurses.

occupational therapists, and respiratory therapists. Even though some of these staff people are employed on a part-time basis, it is important to note that they are on call twenty-four hours a day, as needed. The professional administrative staff say that the advantage of having part-time personnel allows for the fluidity of maintaining hospice service for the patient on a twenty-four hour basis. Additional staff, as well as special therapists and consultants--for example, psychiatrist, nutritionist, pharmacist, and clergy--are utilized on an hourly basis as needed.

Once a patient is deemed appropriate for the hospice program by the clinical evaluation team (physician, nurse, social worker), a nurse and clinical social worker are assigned to complete the nursing and psychosocial assessment based on the medical assessment. A plan of care is then developed by the interdisciplinary caregivers and staff are assigned as needed. The same staff team members continue to see the patient as long as the patient is on the program to provide continuity.

The staffing pattern in the inpatient unit is planned similarly. The home care staff member will continue to visit and provide care in the inpatient unit as though that patient were in his or her home. This constitutes an innovative and unique staffing situation.

The pastoral care department was slow in developing since numerous educational and work sessions were required in order to establish a common approach to spiritual needs and then write policies and procedures to assure integration within the interdisciplinary (IDG) team. The coordinator of pastoral care assigns a clergy of the month to contact all new admissions, attend weekly IDG meetings, and coordinate patient/family needs. In addition, monthly meetings are held to discuss any concerns or problems and present an educational program for members of the group. This sensitive and critical component of care is carefully planned, implemented, and thoughtfully evaluated by Hospice of Pa.'s evaluation process.

Resources Available

The Lady Helena volunteer program developed as needs and appropriate volunteer usage dictated. Volunteers have been involved in every aspect of hospice care from membership on the advisory committee and administrative staff assistance to nursing care, supportive care of the family and patient, and bereavement follow-up. Categories of volunteer service include:

- Direct patient/family care

- Bereavement volunteers

- Receptionists for visitors, mail, telephone

- Public speakers to present program to community organizations

- Clerical assistants assigned to departments for tasks such as: editing, typing, filing, collating, xeroxing, or data collection

- Group workers for mass mailings

- Individual or group workers for updating mailing lists

- Photographers, artists, and writers for special tasks in public information, education, newsletters, brochures, and so on

- Hosts and hostesses for meetings, conferences, workshops

- Hosts and hostesses for social events

- Coordinators for conferences and special events

- Library and resource center workers

- Workers for research of bibliography and audio-visual resources in the community

- Workers for research in community services resources

- Drivers for errands and volunteer transport

- Babysitters for children of volunteers

- Leadership positions in coordinating volunteer teams assigned to a specific job description

- Advisory committee members for planning and evaluation of various aspects of the program

Other community resources were developed through informational meetings held with personnel from Blue Cross/Blue Shield, Medicare, the Department of Welfare, Social Security, Veterans Administration, Meals on Wheels, the Bureau of Vocational Rehabilitation, American Cancer Society, the Early Cancer Detection Center, the Home-Health Agency, the Area Agency on Aging, and the United Way.

Hospice of Pa., Inc. has professional as well as lay volunteers augmenting their program and, in many instances, volunteers perform the following services, as stated in the volunteer manual:

- Reading to the patient

- Acting as senior companions

- Driving the patient to church, physician's office, or to visit relatives

- Marketing

- Respite care

- Personal care

- Chore

- Homemaker

Hospice of Pa., Inc. also utilizes volunteers from "Telespond"--a federally funded service which reimburses the aforementioned volunteers for their time. "Telespond" is an organization which was founded from funds that were intended for care of the elderly, and is funded in part by Volunteers for ACTION, a Federal Volunteer Agency.

Five senior companions from Telespond are assigned daily Monday through Friday from 10 a.m. until 2 p.m. These individuals provide a valuable service to the hospice patient--mainly respite services which allow the family a relief from constant care--and are coordinated by the volunteer director.

Hospice of Pa., Inc. utilizes all existing resources in the community necessary to coordinate care for patients/families, some of which include Cancer Society, Area Agency for Aging, Counseling Center, Department of Welfare, Community Hospital Oncology Program, Volunteers for Action, local universities for educational aspects and student placement as well as many other community agencies.

The hospice supportive care program, consisting of hospice-trained private duty nurses and aides, is augmented by local registries who coordinate closely with the hospice team.

Funding Sources

Varied funding sources are common among the community-based models. In addition to the existing reimbursement system, multiple sources need to be explored.

Since Lady Helena Hospice program was neither operating nor using funds at full capacity until the end of the first year, request was made to and granted by the Department of Health, Education and Welfare (now HHS) Administration on Aging to extend the first year to a fifteen-month period. Referrals to Lady Helena came gradually, giving the staff an opportunity to develop care techniques and establish contact with local physicians and other medical institutions and health caregivers.

Lady Helena Hospice continued to seek sources to supplement the Administration on Aging funding through involvement with United Way agencies, national and local church bodies, private funding agencies, memorial contributions, and gifts. In a projected cost for per diem patient care for two years, as submitted to the United Way, a cost of thirty-six dollars per patient day was established. The patients/families are charged a sliding fee, for nursing service only, which is based on an ability to pay. No one is denied hospice services because of an inability to pay. A patient is admitted to the hospice program on the basis of need. A fee for service scale, based on the family's ability to pay, has been established. Lady Helena also recognized the necessity for home care and hospice certification for the purpose of receiving third party reimbursement--a process which they completed in 1983 and 1984. In addition, their hospice was successful in securing community support for the program. Grants of $10,000 have been received from two dioceses in America. Lady Helena Hospice has been accepted as a member agency of the United Way of that community and is negotiating with the United Way of surrounding communities.

Hospice of Pa., Inc., as a certified hospice and home health agency, receives third-party reimbursement for a majority of services. In addition, a contract for Adult Block Grant Monies covers some counseling, bereavement, and homemaking services. Also, certification as a CORF* allows counseling as well as other covered services.

Additional sources of funding include contributions, grant monies, memorial fund donations, and on-going fundraising activities.

ADVANTAGES AND DISADVANTAGES

Significant to this model is the role which the original administrators take in community, city, and national affairs as board members of the Pennsylvania Hospice Network and Committee Members for the National Hospice Organization.

The coordination and continuity within the community is a major advantage of the community-based model where the expert interdisciplinary hospice team is able to function at any level of care. Lady Helena also has the advantage of initial funding through their parent organization and on-going funding because of their recent certification as a home health agency and a hospice. Services are easily coordinated within the various levels of care in the community because of the specially trained hospice team members' availability to visit in the hospital, home, and nursing home.

Also, the planning for inpatient beds with autonomous administration and control will then fully provide their patients with a holistic approach to hospice care. Hospital and other community resources are available due to formal ties within their implementation of hospice services. Lady Helena Hospice recently set up a hospice unit within a nursing facility offering patients the full gamut of services.

Hospice of Pa., Inc. patients are visited wherever they are--either in their homes, in the hospital, in a nursing home, or other location. The focus, however, is home care. Based on agency policy, home visits are made daily to once weekly depending on the needs of a patient/family as verified by medical record review. A patient may be seen daily by either a registered professional nurse or

---

* There are thirteen eligible services under the Comprehensive Outpatient Rehabilitation Program as discussed earlier.

home health aide for personal and supportive care, by a senior companion for a companion type visit, by a social worker for counseling, supportive care, and financial assistance, by a volunteer for respite type care or transportation to the physician's office, by a physical therapist or speech therapist for rehabilitative services, and by a member of the clergy for spiritual support, a comprehensive approach to utilization of the interdisciplinary team.

Hospice of Pa., Inc.--for the same reasons as Lady Helena--offers a comprehensive coordinated approach to hospice care in the community. Hospice of Pa., Inc. also has an additional advantage: it has a hospice nurse and medical social work coordinator program, a formal liaison with the community hospitals. Autonomous administration allows for full control of the program with flexibility, progress, and easy change when necessary. The specialized interdisciplinary hospice care is able to focus on expert palliative care. As a certified home health agency, the hospice patient can remain in his or her own home with an appropriate support system utilizing the existing reimbursement system.

Again, with inpatient beds, there are institutional resources within their control and a mechanism to implement hospice care policies in an institution.

Advantages of the community-based model include autonomous administration, an administrative team representing various disciplines, a commitment to a program of care by a specialized interdisciplinary care team who focus on expert palliative care, coordination of care within the community itself, a provision that patients can remain in their own homes with an appropriate support system, and cost-effectiveness as demonstrated through an existing reimbursement system.

Disadvantages are minimal and can be easily overcome. They include: (1) limited resources within the program itself such as their own inpatient facility; and (2) a patient's need to have a primary care person to provide care between home visits, which is difficult when individuals live alone.

QUALITY AND THE COMMUNITY-BASED MODEL

Lady Helena Hospice met five out of the nine criteria completely, as shown in Figure 8-1. In relation to direct care, twenty-four hour service was provided, the interdisciplinary team was used, and the patient and the family was seen as a unit of care. Indirectly, administration and coordination were met. In addition, Hospice of Pa. provided volunteer and bereavement services as needed. Pastoral care was provided in 47 percent of the Lady Helena patients studied; volunteer services were provided in 32 percent; pain control according to hospice methods was practiced in 23 percent; and bereavement services were provided in 75 percent of the patients studied. Since the interdisciplinary team was used in 100 percent of the patients perhaps not as many volunteers or clergy were indicated. Lady Helena met five out of the seven new criteria; they do not provide active antitumor therapy and diagnostic tests as components of their program. Not meeting the pain control criterion may have a relationship to the failure to use antitumor therapy, x-rays, and diagnostic tests which perhaps is due to medical practice in that geographic area.

Hospice of Pa., Inc., a separate community organization, met seven out of the nine criteria completely. Pain control methods according to hospice policy were applied in 42 percent of the patients and pastoral care was provided in 46 percent of the patients. The amount of pain control practiced may relate to the amount of patients receiving pastoral care. Hospice of Pa., Inc. met all of the new criteria as shown in Table 8-2. The flexibility relates to the fact that they have their own autonomous administration, allowing fluidity in program planning and development.

ADMINISTRATIVE CONSIDERATIONS

The community-based model without a parent organization meets a significant number of the criteria/standards set up for a pure hospice program with quality services.

The number of criteria met out of the sixteen by each research site is as follows:

Discrete Unit	10
Scattered Bed	9
Home Care-Based	6
Freestanding	9
Community-based with parent organization	10
Community-based without parent organization	14

Table 8-1 and Figures 8-1 and 8-2 provide a comparative summary of sites studied and a summary of criteria met or not met in each research site.

The fact that all patients in all models, regardless of organizational structure, have hospice care available to the patient/family as a unit of care twenty-four hours a day, seven days a week, with coordination by the hospice care team provides a good basis for the *first* step toward quality of care.

Community-based models seek to provide overall coordination of services for the hospice patients and play a major advocacy role in hospice care. This model, through a long-range planning mechanism, implements available services which are identified on the basis of need for patients/families. Central administration provides linkages with acute care facilities, long-term facilities, home care programs, and public health services in both the provision of and planning for hospice care. The community-based model differs from the hospital-based and freestanding models by virtue of its broad-based coordination role using existing community services. However, it is similar in terms of use of a hospice-trained interdisciplinary team integrated into existing services. For this same reason, it is similar to the home care model in that home services are provided by the hospice team in coordination with existing home care services.

To the extent that hospice care programs are able to provide services in a variety of settings, they make it possible for the patient to enter the program without the need to change his or her current setting unless there is a medical necessity to do so. Then patients can enter the program while hospitalized or enter the program while at home and can, without loss of continuity, shift back and forth between settings as necessary. The home care model does not have a formal mechanism for doing this.

The most suitable setting for a particular patient at a particular time depends upon a number of factors; physical condition, the home situation, and his or her attitude toward the illness and family. The input of the members of the interdisciplinary team is important to the decision about where the patient can best receive care. The experience of this author is that most patients and their families prefer to have the patient at home for as much of the terminal illness as possible. Most freestanding hospices with home care programs are handicapped when acute hospital care is necessary. Ideally, there should be facilities available for an intermediate level of care in a nursing home arrangement for those patients who do not have willing and able caregivers in the home or those whose requirements for care are a little more than can be provided in the home but less than necessitate hospitalization--an area discussed in the chapter on the skilled care model.

TABLE 8-1. COMPARATIVE SUMMARY OF SITES STUDIED*

without parent organization	with parent organization	Freestanding	Home Care	Scattered-Bed	Hospital-Based Discrete Unit	RESEARCH SITES	
Community-Based	*Community-Based*						
	●	●	●		●	Executive Director	Administration Supervision (Direct)
●		●			●	RN Director of Pt/family services	
	●			●		RN Pt. Care Coordinator	
			●			Home Health Services Clinical Supervisor	
●	●	●		●	●	Medical Director	
●					●	Director of Social Services	
	●	●		●	●	Director of Volunteers	
		●				Director of Bereavement	
		●				Director of Education	
		●				Director of Evaluation	
●		●				Own	Administration
	●		●	●	●	Parent Organization	
				●	●	Hospital	
●	●		●	●	●	Third Party Reimbursement	Funding Sources
●			●		●	Contributions	
	●					Fee for Service	
	●	●				Federal Grant	
●						Title XX	
●	●		●	●	●	Admission	Written Policies
●	●	●		●		General	
●	●					Patient Coordination	
				●		Nursing	
				●		Consultation	
●	●		●	●	●	Job Description	
●		●	●			Education	
●	●	●	●	●		Volunteer	
●	●	●	●			Bereavement	
		●				Medical Record	
			●			Program Evaluation	
			●		●	Weeks or months	Admission Philosophy (Terminal)
				●		Three to six months	
		●				Six months or less	
	●					Limited	
●						Unlimited	

* Presence - ● or specific number
  Absence - blank

TABLE 8-1. COMPARATIVE SUMMARY OF SITES STUDIED (Cont.) *

RESEARCH SITES

Category	Feature	Community-Based (without parent organization)	Community-Based (with parent organization)	Freestanding	Home Care	Hospital-Based (Scattered-Bed)	Hospital-Based (Discrete Unit)
Admission Philosophy	Palliative Care	●	●	●	●		●
	Chronic Disease	●					
	Primary Care Person Present				●		
	Aggressive Chemotherapy and Radiation Therapy	●					
Programs [Direct]	Inpatient			●		●	●
	Home Care	●	●	●	●	●	
	Education	●	●	●			●
	Volunteer	●	●	●	●	●	●
	Bereavement	●	●	●	●	●	●
Contracts Home Care	Health Department						●
	Visiting Nurse					●	
	Nursing Home			●			
	None	●			●	●	
Team Components (Paid)	Medical		●	●	●		●
	Skilled Nursing	●	●	●	●	●	●
	Licensed Practical Nurse				●		●
	Medical Social Worker	●	●	●	●	●	●
	Health Aide	●			●		●
	Physical/Occupational	●			●		●
	Psychologist				●	●	
	Nutritionist				●	●	
	Speech Therapist	●			●	●	
	Chore Worker				●		
	Clergy			●	●	●	
	Pharmacist				●		
	Homemaker	●				●	
Medical & Statistical Recording System	Expansion of Hospital					●	●
	Expansion of Home Health Service Record				●		
	Own	●	●	●			
Number of Patients	Number Served	99	136	800	53	207	155
	Number Active	42	20	30	18	25	19

* Presence -   ● or specific number
  Absence - blank

TABLE 8-1. COMPARATIVE SUMMARY OF SITES STUDIED (Cont.) *

RESEARCH SITES	Length of Stay		Approximate Cost		Number of Volunteers
	Number of Days	Unknown	Hospital Rate	Cost per Visit	Number
Hospital-Based Discrete Unit	22		●		80
Scattered-Bed	36		●		55
Home Care	45			$35	25
Freestanding	45				190
Community-Based					
with parent organization		●		$85	90
without parent organization	111			$30	100

* Presence - ● or specific number
  Absence - blank

FIGURE 8-1.   SUMMARY OF CRITERIA WHETHER MET OR NOT MET IN EACH RESEARCH SITE *

RESEARCH SITES	24 hr. service	Pain control	Volunteer services	Pastoral care	Interdisciplinary team	Pt/family as unit of care	Administration Administrator	Administration Coordinator	Bereavement
Hospital-Based Discrete Unit	●	◑	●	◔	◐	●	●	●	●
Scattered-Bed	●	◕	◕	◐	◐	●	●	●	●
Home Care	●	◔	◕	○	◔	●	○	●	◕
Freestanding	●	◔	◔	◔	●	●	●	●	◕
Community-Based with parent organization	●	◔	◕	◑	●	●	●	●	◕
without parent organization	●	◑	◑	◑	●	●	●	●	●

*   Percentage is based on the number of patients out of the sample size of thirty in each research site who met the criteria; i.e., approximately fifty percent or fifteen patients in Royal Angelican received services from the interdisciplinary team compared to 100 percent or thirty patients in Seaside, Lady Helena, and Forum.

Legend: ● 100%   ◕ 75%   ◐ 50%   ◔ 25%

FIGURE 8-2. SUMMARY OF NEW CRITERIA WHETHER PRESENT OR ABSENT IN EACH RESEARCH SITE *

RESEARCH SITES	Palliative Care	Anti-tumor Therapy	X-ray and Dx. Studies	Reimbursement	Flexibility and Continuity	Education Program	Evaluation Program
Hospital-Based Discrete Unit	●	○	○	●	●	●	○
Scattered-Bed	●	●	●	●	●	○	○
Home Care	●	○	○	●	●	○	●
Freestanding	●	○	○	○	●	●	●
Community-Based with parent organization	●	○	○	○	●	●	●
without parent organization	●	●	●	●	●	●	●

CRITERIA

* Present - ●
Absent - ○

Chapter 9

Skilled-Nursing Model

MODEL DESCRIPTION

Until recently a review of the literature showed a paucity of information regarding a skilled nursing-based hospice program. In 1982 only eighteen out of 1145 hospice programs were in long-term care facilities (Joint Commission on Accreditation of Hospitals, 1983). For this reason, this model was not included in the research component. In reflecting on the role of nursing homes in care of the terminal patient, we must be alert to the literature which is replete with negative assessments of caregiving in nursing facilities; therefore, we must pose serious questions regarding quality of life in such a setting. References are made to nursing home environments as fostering loss of autonomy and social death.

A hospice-oriented skilled care facility focuses on the dignity of the individual patient and on maintaining quality of life until death. There are many elements of the hospice approach that a patient can experience in such an inpatient environment: a total needs emphasis, increased patient autonomy, open discussion of death, a community ideology, a team orientation that cuts across levels of staff hierarchy, a role blurring of caregivers, utilization of volunteers, focus on patients and families as the unit of care, and mutually beneficial integration of hospice with the outside community (Munley, Powers, and Williamson, 1982).

Personal observations are included here which are pertinent to the discussion of the skilled-nursing model in relation to hospice. This model is a hospice program which functions under the ownership of a long-term care facility.

A TYPICAL SKILLED-NURSING MODEL

Formal and Informal Structure

Hospice can become a component of a comprehensive care center which offers a broad array of institutional and community services under one roof. This "umbrella" approach ensures appropriate, high-quality patient- and family-centered services when and where needed. A continuum of services can be provided consisting of skilled or intermediate care, home care, day care, and transportation services. These services are coordinated with consultation and education services--designed as an interdisciplinary program to provide comprehensive assistance to the terminally ill patient (Kadner and Feldman, 1980). Patients are able to die in their own homes or in a special ten-bed continuing care unit. The program's focus on home care with inpatient service as back-up is made possible by the institution's care continuum.

Some nursing homes in Minnesota have successfully integrated hospice principles into their programs of care. Yet, while many recognize and support the hospice philosophy, few actually utilize specific protocols and policies to see that this philosophy is shared by all staff (Thoreen, 1981).

In the New York City area, Catholic sisters who operate nursing homes have created a unique caring environment wherein patients are encouraged to take care of one another and support one another. These facilities such as Calvary Hospital and St. Rose's are church-related institutions which have sought to care for poor people who have incurable cancer (Rossman, 1979). In these institutions, a cheerful staff brings a spirit of joy into the lives of the terminal patients. A caring, sensitive nurse providing personal care can offer more than medication for pain and can give peace of mind. This significant informal structure within facilities has existed without being labeled a modern hospice.

Forbes Hospice, a member of the Forbes Health System, has eight inpatient beds within their Pittsburgh Skilled Nursing Center as a back-up for the home care program and for other patients in the Forbes Health System who are difficult to manage due to poorly controlled physical symptoms or complex psychosocial problems (Fello, 1984).

An example of a licensed, skilled nursing facility with a hospice unit is the Washington, D.C. Home Hospice, which is a six-bed inpatient unit housed within a large residential nursing home. The Washington Home Hospice program was initially established in cooperation with Georgetown University's home health agency as a source of referral (Reiss, 1982). As a community approach to hospice care, insufficient referrals resulted in expansion of referral sources to include other home health providers and acute hospitals in the general community.

Program Components

A typical hospice component within a skilled nursing facility has the basic philosophy that medical and nonmedical techniques can be used in a variety of settings to provide the terminally ill patient with an alert, pain-free existence, thus preserving to the end a sense of dignity and self-worth. Involvement with the hospice team continues through the period of bereavement.

Responsibility for home care becomes a part of the total health care program lodged within the facility's home care program. One example is a home health agency set up as an alternative to placement in a nursing home or intermediate care facility. The goal of hospice is to have the individual remain at home if at all possible. A hospice inpatient unit is available, therefore, to either prepare the patient for home care or to offer respite care for the patient and family. Round-the-clock coverage is provided at home by a special telephone line to the facility and home visits any time during the day or night as necessary.

The inpatient palliative care is provided in a warm, familiar, home-like environment with twenty-four hour visiting, facilities for on-demand meal preparation, and comfortable accommodations for overnight visitors. Patients are encouraged to bring their own belongings and decorations to personalize the room.

In addition to home care and inpatient services, day care becomes a program component in skilled facilities to temporarily relieve families of their responsibility for caring for relatives at home. The respite provision in the hospice benefit under Medicare allows for only a five-day inpatient stay to relieve families. As an alternative within the skilled model, the day care is a medical and social model delivering needed outpatient treatment, rehabilitation, and psychosocial support. Hospice patients in this day care program also obtain needed socialization and recreational opportunities. Transportation services are also an important part of the hospice day care program.

Educational programs are essential throughout the year to meet the needs and interests of professionals and lay people. Because of the financial implications for educational programs, such program elements often need separate funding through grants. Hospice interdisciplinary team members become true specialists in caring for the terminally ill through an intense training period.

Admission criteria are similar to other models: diagnosis of a terminal illness with a medical prognosis of six months or less; a disease state where palliative care is the only appropriate therapy and patient preference for this level of medical care, along with associated support services and referrals; consent authorization by the patient's primary physician; and presence of a primary care person who assumes responsibility for the patients' care at home.

Staffing Patterns

The skilled-nursing hospice becomes a family-centered service which is provided by a specially trained staff of professionals and volunteers. Staff consists of physicians, nursing personnel, social workers, rehabilitation therapists, recreationists, psychologist, dietician, clinical pharmacologist, clergyman, clerical workers, and volunteers.

Because of the intensive nature of care provided to hospice patients and their families, there is often a higher staff per patient ratio than would commonly be found in nursing homes or hospitals. Nursing services in a hospice unit are often delivered at the level of an intensive care unit in a hospital or eight hours of care per patient per day; whereas, a traditional skilled-nursing facility requires total nursing and nurse's aide personnel to be 1.40 hours per patient from 7 a.m. to 9 p.m. and .50 hours per patient from 9 p.m. to 7 a.m. Hospice also provides a framework to ensure a twenty-four hour, seven-day-a-week, on-call physician availability including home visits and eight hour-a-day on-site medical staff coverage. A skilled-nursing facility has a physician available by phone twenty-four hours per day, available to respond promptly to an emergency, and an alternate physician for coverage whenever necessary (Johnson-Hurzeler, Barnum, and Abbott, 1983).

Staff morale must be considered in that nurses and other staff responsible for nonhospice patients may perceive the hospice unit, its staff, and its patients as receiving "most-favored" treatment. Here the educational program and staff and patient support groups are essential. Staff and patient preparation for a new hospice program is critical. Time must be spent by planners, supervisory, and administrative personnel to clearly create a positive attitude among caregivers throughout the entire facility.

Resources Available

The use of volunteers in the skilled-nursing model makes possible the provision of personalized services which would otherwise be financially prohibitive if professionals had to be hired. The volunteer component needs to be expanded to include direct caregiving. Here again the volunteer training through educational sessions must be done thoughtfully and comprehensively. Volunteers can easily perform such activities as washing the patient's hair, helping the patient write letters, and seeing that the patient is close to the outdoors either through a window or on a patio to enjoy nature and people. The touching needs of patients can be carried out by volunteers or staff: holding hands, stroking the patient's arm, other such continual personal reassurances to the dying patient which transmit love and caring. A skilled-nursing facility has a personal care area where patients can go for haircuts or shampoos and sets--an already existing resource not as readily available in any other hospice model.

Use of community resources and establishment of coordinated services, affiliations, and linkages is important to the program's success and should result in an excellent public relations mechanism along with an image of excellence in the community--a quality care component.

Funding Sources

Reimbursement rates in nursing homes present a financing problem, the main problem being that of staffing. Hospice care requires a higher staffing ratio than the traditional nursing home. The cost of one hospice program based at a nursing home in Washington, D.C. is $176 per day--well above average reimbursement rates for skilled nursing care (Healy, 1980). At least for the inpatient component of hospice programs, hospital-based hospices are able to get more reimbursement than nursing homes for the more comprehensive nursing care needed by terminal patients.

Yet, with a comprehensive program which includes volunteers and students, a skilled-nursing facility is a more appropriate level of care at a more reasonable cost. Hospice providers are concerned about programs labeled "hospice" which may offer a minimal amount of care while receiving reimbursement at the full rate.

Hospice representatives must seek demonstration and pilot projects with varied funding sources. Third-party payors such as Blue Cross Plans, Group Plans, Health Maintenance Organizations (HMO), Preferred Provider Organizations (PPO), and other commercial insurers are forthcoming reimbursement sources.

ADVANTAGES AND DISADVANTAGES

Probably the major advantage of a skilled nursing model is cost-effectiveness since hospice inpatient services can be provided in a lower-cost inpatient-skilled facility. The conversion of skilled-facility beds into special hospice units is a way of avoiding capital costs associated with construction of a new freestanding hospice facility.

Skilled-nursing facilities can be ideally suited for adaptation to hospice programs since they are less technology-intensive settings, and generally more home-like and accessible than hospitals. On the other hand, a disadvantage may be the lack of full-time supportive services considered necessary to render proper hospice care; skilled facilities would, therefore, have to upgrade their staffing patterns to accommodate the hospice role.

Nursing homes can create a positive environment concerning death and dying since residents can support each other as they face death and often create an open communication policy among staff and residents.

The Minnesota study revealed that although nursing homes tend to recognize and meet the needs of the dying residents and their families, they reflect a lack of specific protocols, policies, practices, and agreements with other providers that are geared toward meeting these needs (Thoreen, 1981).

Skilled-nursing facilities have begun to see a growing acceptance of long-term care as an integral part of the health care delivery system. There has been a marked improvement in the quality of care provided in skilled-nursing facilities with increasing involvement of the facility and the community in an interrelationship. The long-term care administrator's desk manual now includes a section on community relations, discussing programs and methods requiring an ongoing commitment and administrative support (Miller, 1982), which is certainly conducive to creation of a hospice unit.

QUALITY AND THE SKILLED-NURSING MODEL

Nursing homes can adopt and apply certain components of a hospice program with ease but it is unlikely that homes will be able to implement full-fledged hospice programs based on all quality criteria without maximum effort and some experience. Certain quality criteria such as meeting the total bereavement needs of families, providing home care, and actively involving physicians in interdisciplinary teamwork may not be realistic for the average long-term care facility.

Formal consulting and service arrangements should be developed between hospice programs and other community services and nursing homes in order to achieve continuity and flexibility of services. Autonomous administration for the hospice beds within a skilled facility is an important characteristic to retain. In addition, the facility must be committed to the extension of the interdisciplinary team to include all areas of expertise, and time must be allowed for regular meetings of the IDG team.

The Washington Home Hospice added a full-time administrator for the hospice unit in order to maintain a more focused administrative approach and to oversee the admissions process. This permitted more effective liaison with referring providers, and created an opportunity to coordinate educational sessions for nonhospice staff at the Home in order to improve morale and foster better staff relationships (Wilson, Blosse, Tucker, and Spector, 1983).

The importance of a quality educational program for nursing home administrators and their staff is an important step in the process of implementing hospice programs within skilled facilities. Sensitizing health care professionals and volunteers through education about the special needs of these persons is an important focus. Many nursing home patients and hospice-type patients have similar needs.

In many ways the skilled-nursing model can influence the improvement of the total health care system in providing a special place and specially-trained persons for the chronically and terminally ill. It appears to be an appropriate setting as an extension of existing home health care services and services to bereaved families.

ADMINISTRATIVE CONSIDERATIONS

Nursing home administrators need to examine hospice principles and services, then study which best meet the needs of their patients. They should recognize the areas of concern which must be addressed if implementation of hospice principles seem appropriate and feasible. Administrators must fully understand and train staff in the philosophical foundations of hospice care and assure that the pure aspects of hospice are integrated into the programs and practices of the home. Again, education becomes an important component and a primary endeavor for a successful hospice program within their facility. From both a planning and financial perspective, a skilled-nursing model can make innovative use of existing services and widen the range of care. At the same time, this minimizes costly service duplication and fragmentation in the community; it certainly eliminates capital and start-up costs, and reduces ongoing costs.

This model must also provide a home care component with a continuum of care through staffing methods to bridge the transfer from inpatient care to home care and vice versa. Administration must provide for bereavement needs of family and friends with trained staff to identify pathological grief reactions and to refer to proper community resources when necessary.

Skilled-nursing administrators who are seeking to develop a system of hospice care should develop well-defined protocols for patient admission assessment, care evaluation, and transfer processes to avoid inappropriate admissions and levels of service. Equally important are clearly defined administrative and operational policies for the hospice unit within the existing health service entity.

Organizationally, hospice care may be more comfortably located in a nursing home, where goals relate to rehabilitation or custodial care rather than cure. The time has come, perhaps, to adapt humanizing hospice principles of care to the nursing home model by applying increased ingenuity and innovativeness to a hospice unit within the facility.

REFERENCES

Fello, Maryanne. 1984. Interview with Author. Forbes Hospice, July.

Healy, William. (1980). Hospice. What Is It? *American Health Care Association Journal* (July):51-56.

Johnson-Hurzeler, Rosemary, Evelyn Barnum, and John Abbott. (1983). Hospice: The Beginning Or The End? The Impact of TEFRA on Hospice Care In The United States. *University of Bridgeport Law Review* 5(1):69-105.

Joint Commission on Accreditation of Hospitals. (1983). *JCAH Hospice Project*. Chicago.

Kadner, Dennis L., and Eli S. Feldman. (1980). Hospice as Part of the Care Continuum in a Comprehensive Geriatric Center. *The Journal of Long-Term Care Administration* 8:43-49.

Miller, Dulcy B. (1982). *Long Term Care Administrator's Desk Manual.* New York: Panel Publishers, Inc.

Munley, Anne, Cynthia S. Powers, and John B. Williamson. (1982). Humanizing Nursing Home Environments: The Relevance of Hospice Principles. *International Journal on Aging and Human Development.* 15(4):263-283.

Reiss, Kay. (1982). *Hospice Care: A Federal Role?* Congressional Research Service, Library of Congress, Report No. 82-49 EPW, March 22nd.

Rossman, Parker. (1979). *Hospice.* New York: Fawcett Columbine.

Thoreen, Peter W. (1981). *Death, Dying and Terminal Care: Issues Faced By The Long-Term Care Facility.* Minneapolis, MN: Long-Term Care Committee of the Minnesota Coalition for Terminal Care, Inc.

Wilson, Barry P., Raymond W. Blosse, Jon L. Tucker, and Kristin K. Spector. (1983). Hospice Care: Perspectives On A Blue Cross Plan's Community Pilot Program. Washington, DC: Blue Cross/Blue Shield Association.

Chapter 10

Hospice Models: A Comparative View

Common themes present themselves in all models discussed in Chapters 5 through 8. The philosophy underlying each hospice program emphasizes palliative medical and social care for the terminally ill patient with emphasis on improving the quality of life for the patient and family. The goals are to allow the patient to live at home in his customary environment as long as appropriate and to support the family in caring for the patient. Support continues in all models to help them bridge the void left when a loved one dies.

Almost all hospice organizations from their inception have had to adapt to varying circumstances and conditions such as demographic statistics, community attitudes, and community planning. The salient features of all models can be compared. All of the research on the various hospice sites provide in some way the following components:

Philosophical goals. In all models the patient and family are the raison d'etre for the hospice program. According to a review of policy documents, the patient and family participate in the decisions and caregiving which enables the patient and family to live according to their "style" and with the dignity and respect due all human beings until the moment of the patient's death. With similar philosophy each hospice model considers the patient and the family together in providing services. All models prefer that there be a primary caregiver available to the patient.

Parent organization. The hospital-based and home care model have a distinct parent organization unlike the freestanding and the community model. The parent organization not only provides administration but also funding support for these organizations.

Funding mechanism. Funding sources vary among the models. Seawing Hospice is the only site which did not receive third-party reimbursement since they functioned under the NCI grant. A fee-for-service scale exists only in the community model. Lady Helena has utilized this fee scale yet remained flexible in providing services regardless of the patient/family ability to pay. One program, Hospice of Pa., Inc., provides services under Title XX* for homemaking and counseling, a resource other hospices are now pursuing. Based on interviews with site administrators regarding funding, the annual budgets vary greatly. Budgets of the hospital-based model research sites were between $100,000 to $150,000 compared to one community model site which had a budget of approximately $55,000. The operating budget of the freestanding model based on the NCI Grant was approximately $660,000. The home care model was estimated at $125,000 based on the overall agency budget.

Professional training of administrator. The hospital-based sites function under the hospital administrator. The inpatient hospice unit site also has a hospice administrator with a doctorate in philosophy responsible to the overall hospital administration. Each hospital model has a registered nurse as a patient care coordinator. The freestanding model has a full-time administrator with a masters degree in public health as well as a director of nursing with a bachelor of science degree in nursing. Currently this model, having moved into a hospital setting, has a registered nurse as a patient care coordinator.

The home care model utilizes the home health agency executive director, a professional nurse as hospice administrator, and the home health agency registered nurse clinical supervisor for overall supervision. A registered nurse specialist in terminal illness coordinates the hospice team. The community-based model represented by two research sites differ in administrator credentials. Lady Helena, who received funding from Administration on Aging, has an individual with a masters degree in rehabilitation counseling administering the agency and a registered nurse coordinating patient services. Hospice of Pa., with limited start-up funding, uses a registered professional nurse administrator, a medical social worker as a chief executive officer, and full-time registered professional nurse supervisors/coordinators in collaboration with a medical social work supervisor/coordinator.

Organizational structure. The services of the hospice program are coordinated under a central administration to optimize utilization of services and resources. Programs in all models are under medical direction of an oncologist on a staff or consultant basis. The hospital-based inpatient unit and freestanding institution have a staff oncologist available as needed, whereas the remaining sites utilize the oncologist on a consultant basis. There are formal and/or written arrangements for the continuing involvement of the attending physicians. All models recognize the need to accommodate the desires of the attending physicians.

---

* Title XX is now known as Adult Block Grants.

All the models have policy and procedure manuals, as well as record-keeping systems, statistical report formats, personnel policies, and job descriptions. These are all in various stages of development with all administrators recognizing the need for well-written and up-to-date documents as their program changes. The home care model has a well-stated program evaluation in keeping with the required regulations for certification. This appears to be a component that will be further developed in the other models as the programs become well established. Quality assurance efforts currently reflect the existing quality assurance programs in the hospital and home care models and Hospice of Pa. (a community model with home health agency certification); that is, the Joint Commission on Accreditation of Hospitals (JCAH) requires that all hospices have a mechanism for assuring quality of care as well as the Federal Conditions for Participation for home health certification. Other quality assurance efforts reflect the embryonic state of the art.

Referral process. According to written agency policy all models utilize existing resources in the community for appropriate referrals. The hospice programs studied have not duplicated traditional programs of care. The home care and community-based models have in-place referral mechanisms to inpatient facilities for patients requiring hospitalization. Hospice staff have permission to follow their patients in the hospitals to provide continuity of psychosocial support and to work with hospital staff in appropriate pain and symptom control. Hospital discharge planners and social workers are now attending hospice conferences to assure continuity between home, hospital and home.

Admission process. As revealed in the written admission policies, admission criteria vary among the models. All sites except Hospice of Pa. state a prognosis of weeks to months. Hospice of Pa. has an unlimited prognosis; they accept patients with chronic illnesses and also those patients receiving active chemotherapy and radiation therapy.

Approval of attending physician. All models require a signed informed consent form from the patient/family who are informed that they are part of the team and they can leave the program if they desire without any repercussions in the care they will receive. Admission criteria are similar as described in all models except the community-based. Hospice of Pa. expanded their admission criteria to include patients/families with a longer prognosis and unrestricted diagnoses, unlike the freestanding model which is limited to the diagnosis of cancer. Because of the expanded admission criteria at Hospice of Pa. and an effort to encourage referrals at the point of diagnosis the number of diagnostic studies and use of therapeutic measures are greater. Their goal is toward early intervention so that the patient/family never get to the point where the pathology overwhelms them; they are already in the support system.

In other research sites, symptom control is accomplished with the use of a minimum of diagnostic studies and invasive therapeutic measures. In all models, symptoms are considered to include psychosocial problems, as well as physical complaints. Personnel from all models, however, share the feeling that an extremely short life expectancy also presents a problem. The patient who dies within a day or so of entering the program almost invariably gains little or nothing from participation while using some of the limited resources of the program. The GAO (1979) reports that in their review of hospices in the United States, 13 hospices out of the 59 operating hospices were able to provide statistics on the patient's average length of participation in the program, which ranged from 13.9 to 105 days.* For the fifteen hospices with inpatient facilities that reported average length of inpatient stay data, it averaged twenty days, ranging from 8 to 60 days. The hospice with the 60-day average length of stay reports that once patients are admitted to the inpatient facility, they usually remain until they die. The inpatient discrete unit research site was able to provide some detailed statistics on length of stay for 196 patients shown in Table 10-2.

TABLE 10-1. NUMBER OF PATIENTS BY LENGTH OF STAY IN EACH LOCATION (TOTAL DAYS)

Number of Days	Inpatient	Home	Hospital, Other	Total for Program	
				Number	Percent
None	22	92	177		
1-9	112	39	15	73	37%
10-29	47	33	2	62	32%
30-59	11	15	2	33	17%
60-89	1	8	0	11	5%
90+	2	9	0	17	9%
TOTAL PATIENTS	195	196	196	196	100%

Thirty-seven percent of the patients had a length of stay of less than 9 days at the inpatient discrete unit and 32 percent between 10 and 29 days. The scattered-bed research site, according to the registered professional nurse coordinator, had an average length of stay of 36 days compared to the freestanding model whose administrator cited theirs at 45 days. The community-

---

* This figure does not mean average length of stay in an inpatient facility, but includes both home and inpatient care. It does not include the length of time patients' family members participate in the program after patients' deaths.

based and the home care model statistics also showed an average length of stay of 45 days.

Team composition. Components of the team have variance between research sites as evidenced during interviews with the nurse coordinators. A psychologist is used in two sites--freestanding and scattered-bed models. Utilization of the clergy varies also. The inpatient facilities have a chaplain available at all times. Lady Helena, the community-based model and Seawing, the freestanding model both have a paid chaplain as a member of the team. A nutritionist is used as a consultant in three research sites--home care, community-based (Hospice of Pa.) and freestanding. The hospital-based hospice programs have nutritionists accessible from the hospital who are not hospice staff. The freestanding hospice has a paid staff pharmacist who acts as a consultant. Other sites have access to a pharmacist as the need arises. Hospice of Pa., Inc. has a volunteer pharmacist on the professional advisory board who is available when needed. Volunteers are members of the team but are used for a variety of reasons within the hospice programs.

The approach within each model is humanistic in the sense that they direct attention to the ''whole patient'' and draw upon the whole armamentarium of medical care through the use of an interdisciplinary team.

Use of volunteers. In each research site there are formal and written guidelines for recruitment, training, selection, supervision, continuing education, and performance evaluation. The number of volunteers recruited is based on the need of each individual patient/family caseload. Many hospice administrators state that they cannot take all of the volunteers who approach them. The selection process for volunteers is well-organized in all models based on review of the volunteer policy manuals. The screening and on-going coordination of volunteer services with the hospice care team is a careful process within each model to prevent both volunteer and staff stress reactions. Mutual sharing and assistance among volunteers and members of the hospice care team provide effective weapons in the prevention of harmful stress reactions. On-going recruitment and training of volunteers within each model provide a core of volunteers to draw upon due to the inevitable attrition which normally takes place within any volunteer program. It is the variety of work that makes hospice volunteerism so special. Each hospice model provides for leaves of absence for volunteers who request them, and volunteers are allowed to switch over to nonpatient-care work if they wish. Due to funding limitations, volunteers frequently cover the office, answering the telephone and coordinating messages. Other volunteers function as members of the team, providing services to patients. Volunteer services differ according to the needs of each model. A number of hospice programs have expanded the volunteer role in the bereavement program; some are now handled primarily through volunteers. A recent telephone interview with the director of Lady Helena Hospice revealed that due to the high cost of hospice services (85 dollars a visit), they were planning to change their bereavement program so that most of the time spent would be with volunteers. In fact, they were looking to other programs for guidance in developing a volunteers bereavement program. All the models offer the volunteer the choice of nonhome care or noncaregiving roles; the director of volunteers can sometimes sense that the volunteer is not ready for direct care or for the particular demands of work in patients' homes.

Patient care setting. In the hospital-based and freestanding models with inpatient facilities, the same elements exist as for home care, complete with twenty-four hour visiting privileges, rooms for families to spend the night, and accommodations made for pets to visit. There are also kitchens equipped for families to prepare meals, which helps the patients and their families continue their close relationship.

Caseload variance. The caseload varied from site to site. Initially, when selected, each hospice administrator claimed an average caseload of 30 living patients and this remained fairly constant. The current average caseload ranges from 20 to 40 in the hospital-based and between 25 and 30 in the freestanding sites. The community models sites differed--Lady Helena had twenty to twenty-five patients and Hospice of Pa., had over 100. This increase at Hospice of Pa. was reportedly due to certification and expansion of admission criteria and ongoing funding sources.

This comparative summary provides any community and hospice administrator with information on the strengths and weaknesses within each model and pertinent observations regarding numerous aspects of hospice care.

REFERENCES

U.S. General Accounting Office. (1979). *Hospice Care--A Growing Concept In The United States.* HRD-79-50, March 6 .

PART III

IMPLICATIONS FOR THE FUTURE

Chapter 11

Trends, Issues, and Opportunities

As we have seen, hospice can be a program, a building, a concept, or a philosophy; hospice care encompasses inpatient care, outpatient care, home care, day care, education, bereavement services, and research. Hospice respects the dying person's experience and allows the individual to end his or her days in harmony and with dignity.

Hospice is a framework for a curriculum that interfaces medical care with education. Seguine (1983) notes that hospice embodies an interdisciplinary knowledge base that integrates the psychomotor, cognitive, and affective domains of learning. Included within this spectrum would be learning experiences related to death education, psychology of dying, bioethics, counseling of dying patients, administration and organization of hospice programs, social gerontology, geropsychiatry, exercise modules, occupational therapy, psychosocial dynamics of the grief continuum, pharmacopoeia of pain, and others.

The Challenge of Change: Competition or Cooperation

Hospice is creative and innovative, although power politics, varied community responses, and competition have, at times, presented barriers to change. Many people don't want to understand hospice as an important new component within the system which extends beyond any traditional care program. A well-educated board member of a traditional visiting nurse association asks, "Is hospice trying to take us over?"; the questioner fails to understand the fact that the terminal and the chronic patient need to survive with a *special kind of care*. To this particular board member, hospice means competition.

Hospice directly confronts the challenge of change and conflict within the health care delivery system. Starr (1982) reminds us that the dream of reason does not take the desire for power into account. Nevertheless, hospice can become a vehicle toward communication for various groups and--more important--may reestablish death as a home-based event that includes professional medical support systems (Ward, 1978).

The hospice movement brings many challenges to health care practitioners and administrators. Hospice representatives advocate high-quality care that stresses palliation over technology for the terminal patient. Hospice presents an opportunity certainly for the incorporation of research with a commitment for care; data collection can be a useful management tool.

Rediscovering the importance of fulfilling human relationships and their role in well-being is certainly an objective of the interdisciplinary team. Knowledge of other cultures and the effective handling of symptom control are crucial components of hospice care.

Legislation has opened up many opportunities for hospice care. Hospice would be well-served and would be better able to serve its clientele as a Health Maintenance Organization provider and as a preferred provider. Hospice standards can only improve if the IDG team is an absolute nonnegotiable feature, and if there is continuity with home care after hospital care. The health care system no longer needs to revolve around rehabilitation and acute care. For the first time, family involvement is a prime feature of health care. Central autonomous administration within a hospice program allows flexibility and continuity, and eliminates fragmentation.

Hospice has become an alternate health care delivery system which reflects trends within the total health care system. One example is the day care program which is a center and facility designed to accommodate impaired or frail individuals during daytime hours. It provides a safe, protected environment indoors and outdoors, personal care facilities, health care and maintenance services including therapies, monitoring and education, programmed social and physical activities, and a relief or respite for working families and those who provide twenty-four hour care. This is, in fact, an important component of any hospice program model.

Relationship to the Medical Care System

Among those of us who have looked carefully at hospice care, one of the principal concerns has been the relationship between hospice care in particular and medical care in general. There are innumerable forms which this relationship could take. At one extreme is the frightening prospect of a totally separate system for the care of the terminally ill, entirely outside of and completely unrelated to the rest of health care. Zimmerman (1981) states that serious hospice workers would be less than realistic if they considered unthinkable the development of a cult-like phenomenon for the care of the terminally ill. At the opposite extreme is the thought that within the hospice concept are the seeds of a healthy self-destruction, in the course of which hospice care would become completely amalgamated into general medical care perfusing many of its precepts into the management of acutely ill patients. In truth, it is improbable that the future will take us to either of these extremes. As is often the case, the central part of the spectrum seems not only more sensible, but also more likely.

A number of features of the care of the terminally ill suggest that management of such patients will, in some respects be a specialty, but one that fits comfortably into the framework of the traditional medical care system. The unique problems faced by the dying are of such a nature as to merit the special attention of certain physicians. There will always be a sizable number of physicians who, confronted with patients who reach the stage of terminal disease, do not, for one reason or another, wish to be responsible for the continuing care of the patient. Surgeons, radiotherapists, and oncologists are particularly likely to fall in this group. Their reasons for not wishing to continue in the care of the patient are usually sound and we would be prudent to honor them. Thus the need to provide terminal care and the need to find means to improve that terminal care will direct us toward the development of a specialty in the care of the terminally ill. Accordingly, Balfour Mount, M.D. argues that more physician involvement is essential to provide the level and quality of care intended for hospital patients. In a recent interview with an American Hospital Association representative, he stated: "The complex medical problems facing these patients demand intensive physician involvement if symptoms are to be accurately assessed and completely controlled, and the road thus cleared to optimal psychosocial and spiritual intervention. Palliative care services must never become an excuse for mediocrity in medical management." (American Hospital Association, 1984).

The Question of Standards: Methods of Measurement

The matters of standards and certification deserve considerable attention and unquestionably will continue to do so in the years ahead. Care of the terminally ill and hospice care are not alone in this scrutiny. However, because these areas are identifiable as newcomers to the health care arena because they possess certain features that are particularly prone to abuse, representatives from these specialties will have to deal with some important issues.

Use of the term hospice also presents some problems. Certification as a hospice program under the Medicare benefit as discussed earlier raises many questions in hospice development. A slow pace continues for hospice Medicare applications. Hospital-based hospices and coalition models seem to be shying away from Medicare hospice benefits because of perceived inadequate levels of payment and particularly problematic core services requirements.

The National Hospice Organization has taken the initiative in developing standards for hospices. Several considerations must be borne in mind as standards for hospice care are formulated--particularly on the state level. As in all areas of medical care, the establishment of standards must not become an impediment to progress. It is particularly important in hospice care that there be enough flexibility to permit diversity and innovation. It is equally important that the initiative for setting and enforcing standards remain with those in the field of hospice care, rather than in the hands of government agencies. As discussed earlier in Part I, the Joint Commission on Accreditation of Hospitals conducts voluntary accreditation surveys by a JCAH hospice surveyor with first-hand knowledge of hospice programs by reviewing the program for compliance with JCAH's national hospice care standards. Kellogg Foundation awarded monies to JCAH to develop, in cooperation with NHO, quality standards of hospice care; this project led to the national voluntary accreditation program. Cooperation between JCAH and NHO agencies can strengthen the accreditation process as it relates to the care of the terminally ill.

In addition to certification or accreditation of hospices, there is the issue of assessing the quality of care within hospices. JCAH requires that all hospitals have a mechanism for assuring quality of care. It is important that each hospital that treats terminally ill patients apply these mechanisms to the evaluation of care of those patients whether or not it has a hospice care program. Quality assurance through audit can be a demanding and time-consuming process, but hospital-affiliated hospice programs should be certain that they are included in the medical care evaluation process in the hospital. This requires the setting of criteria and the review of data.

Miccio (1984) advocates a practical approach to quality assurance for hospice reduced to its most uncomplicated level. Quality assurance has become an organizational tenet, fundamental to quality health care and accreditation. It has gone through a metamorphosis, being transformed from the structured diagnosis-based audits to a management information system and a method for evaluation of the process of care and for resolution of problems.

An early step which will be a particularly challenging one will involve the development of measurement tools. The objective of hospice care is the control of symptoms in the broadest sense of that term. Symptoms, whether physical or psychological, are by their nature subjective. Measurement of subjective phenomena is difficult, but not impossible. Hospice workers, who have the advantage of already being geared to an interdisciplinary approach, must be ready to draw upon a variety of fields in which subjective factors are measured. Techniques applicable to hospice patients have already been developed; the time has come for their application. The capacity to assess the degree of relief of pain, weakness, nausea, anxiety and depression will open important vistas for hospice care (Zimmerman, 1981).

Measurement tools that relate not to symptom relief but to the organization and cost of hospice care need to be developed. Some new techniques for quantification of personnel time and program component costs should be developed. Many of these techniques already exist and only need to be applied, perhaps with some modification (Zimmerman, 1981).

As measurement tools are developed they can and should be applied by hospice workers to study a number of problems. There clearly needs to be comparison of hospice care with other forms of care for the terminally ill. Until now, efforts to promote the development of hospice care have hinged largely on subjective descriptions and anecdotes. Those who remain skeptical have the right to demand more information. Hospice should be ready to provide them with the data.

The Need for Research

A new study published in the British medical journal, *The Lancet*, shows that hospice improves even conventional care of terminally ill patients. The study, reviewed by NHO's research and evaluation committee, chaired by Barrie R. Cassileth, was conducted at a Los Angeles hospital where differences were explored in pain control, psychological symptoms, and satisfaction with care between hospice and nonhospice patients. "Patients assigned to hospice versus standard treatment expressed greater satisfaction with their care. However, the two patient groups did not differ on the other aspects of care studied. An informal transfer of information and technique from hospice to nonhospice staff appears to have resulted in improved care for nonhospice patients" (NHO, 1984).

There is even greater need, however, for the application of further research techniques within hospice care; there is a need for the comparison of various techniques of hospice care. We must apply acceptable measurement tools to the study of alternative methods of treatment of symptoms. It is when this is done that we can begin to reap the full fruits of what hospice care has to offer.

We also need to apply our measurement tools to the relative merits of different organizational structures within hospice care. It is through such study that we can make further and more rational decisions regarding the selection of a model of hospice care for a given community.

An area to which some investigative effort should be directed is the question of the effect of hospice care on the quantity of life. Since the overall goal of a program for the care of the terminally ill is the expansion of both the quantity and quality of life, the impact of various treatment measures on duration of survival can be useful information in making clinical decisions. The effect of various forms of therapy on survival duration has, of course, a financial as well as clinical dimension; knowledge about this can be helpful (Zimmerman, 1981).

The Involvement of Educational Institutions

One interesting and anomalous feature of hospice care is that, in England and in the United States, it has developed so largely outside our academic institutions. This is surprising because it has been so seldom in the last several decades that medicine has seen something as valuable and with as much potential impact as hospice care develop with so little input from major medical centers and universities. Notwithstanding the closer relationship of Canadian hospices or palliative care programs to medical schools and recognizing the role of a few institutions such as Georgetown University, the lack of involvement on the part of American teaching centers has been striking (Zimmerman, 1981). However, Riverside Hospice in New Jersey was fortunate in that the office of Consumer Health Education, Department of Environmental and Community Medicine, and the College of Medicine and Dentistry of New Jersey-Rutgers Medical School assisted in the development and evaluation of four training manuals:

- *Hospice Volunteers: A Guide for Training* (1980)

- *Bereavement: A Guide for Training* (1981)

- *Hospice: A Guide for Professional Training* (1982)

- *Pain Control in Advanced Cancer Patients: A Guide for Professional Training* (1982)*

The desirability of university involvement in hospice care in the future is an important focus. Hospice administrators need the interest, support, and involvement of the academic institution. University medical centers are the repositories of resources which hospices need. They possess educational capabilities; it is through the introduction of medical students and house officers to hospice care as a part of the fabric of medical practice that we can hope to see the widespread application of hospice principles to the terminally ill. University medical centers have the research capacity, expertise, and experience which can be so valuable to the future care of the terminally ill. This is not to suggest that every university hospital needs to open a hospice care unit. There are various means by which academic centers can become involved in hospice care; such involvement would be to the advantage of both the universities and hospices. Put another way, academic institutions and major medical centers possess talents and a stature in our society which can only be ignored at some peril (Zimmerman, 1981).

Summary of Key Issues

The salient issues in hospice care are, to a large extent, those of our health care system in general. An overriding concern is the need to integrate the social components of care into the total health system. Emphasis on care--controlling symptoms and enhancing the quality of remaining life--not cure, is characteristic of the hospice approach. Other key issues include the following:

---

*This manual was developed jointly by the Office of Consumer Health Education, College of Medicine and Dentistry of New Jersey-Rutgers Medical School, and Calvary Hospital, Bronx, New York.

- Patient/family control versus professional control, including involvement of patients and families in all aspects of treatment decisions that affect them.

- The assurance of a continuum of care that includes bereavement counseling for families.

- Flexible and creative use of resources--professional, volunteer, familial, community-based, and institutional.

- Multiple access to care other than via the acute care system.

- Reassessment of sociomedical values, including the use of drugs and of "heroic" measures to prolong life.

- Redefinition of traditional professional roles and responsibilities, including the concept of the treatment "team".

- Recognition of the need for specialized training for all those involved in working with dying patients and their families (National Association of Social Work, 1981).

Hospice care providers are reminded that continued hard work is needed to meet the challenge of establishing hospice care as a credible and competent health care service.

On the basis of experience thus far it would appear that the approach embodied in the philosophy and practice of hospice care offers the potential for improved care of the terminally ill at a reasonable cost. Hospice programs are likely to increase in numbers and in sophistication. Both the art and science of hospice care will grow with experience. Hospice care can reach its full potential as it becomes an integral part of our medical care system. The needs of dying patients and their loved ones demand no less (Zimmerman, 1981).

In 1981 the W.K. Kellogg Foundation gave NHO a grant of $611,700 to be used over a three-year period for the education and training of hospice personnel. This grant, according to Magno (1981), will be used to improve the quality of hospice care in the United States by providing training opportunities and promoting the *exchange of ideas* among hospice caregivers, administrators, trustees, and volunteers. In addition, the Kellogg Foundation awarded a two-year, $179,504 grant to the American Medical Association in Chicago to design, test, evaluate, and disseminate a system for obtaining and maintaining quality hospice medical records.

It is important to note here that hospice care is not appropriate for everyone. As a community designs a hospice care program, it must look at its own particular circumstances. The program should be tailored to the needs of the specific community, with the research findings regarding its organization and administration kept in mind.

There are many unanswered questions regarding hospice care in the future. Future studies might include a comprehensive look at the impact of hospice care in the various models on staff, patient, and families. It seems that expectations for both care and the behavior of the terminal patient in hospice lack clarity. Future research should examine patterns of adaptation among nurses and patients/families in hospice models.

Assessing the success of symptom and pain relief in a hospice program is difficult. Since symptoms are by definition subjective, there are difficulties in measuring them and documenting changes in them. The development of techniques that will permit objective assessment of results is one of the challenges for the future, for it is in this way that we will be able to evaluate alternative approaches. It is even more difficult, of course, to assess the results of hospice team efforts in dealing with psychological and social problems and in providing spiritual support (Zimmerman, 1981).

Finally, program evaluation research should be developed to enable hospice administrators to make important decisions regarding their services.

As a result of the National Cancer Institute's (NCI) cost analysis study of three freestanding programs-- Hillhaven Hospice, Kaiser-Permanente Hospice, and Riverside Hospice--recommendations for future study are: (1) Studies comparing total costs for hospice and nonhospice patients, and (2) studies to determine which hospice models are more cost-effective without compromising program purposes and goals. NCI's study suggests that, in some cases, freestanding comprehensive hospice services may *not* be cost-effective because of the large staff requirements and patient load limitations. It is generally desirable to have hospices located in proximity to patients; however, in some areas the potential patient population is not large enough to warrant a separate hospice.

Studies also need to be developed to determine outcomes of hospice care based on defined criteria, standards, objectives, and goals; for example, what should be the level of family function six weeks after death of a loved one as a result of bereavement counseling. From this exploratory study one can hypothesize some relationship between and among variables. Specific studies should be performed to determine the benefits of differing staff levels, staff mix, and use of volunteers. Future research should include a national sample to determine outcomes of hospice care through assessment, patient/family analysis, implementation, and evaluation.

Hospice programs are still in their infancy with a new enthusiasm which may change in their growth to adulthood, a caveat from experiences among hospice programs. Neophyte organizations need guidance through the labyrinth of state and federal regulations and bureaucracies.

In July 1984, NHO made a move to study the issues facing hospices that are volunteer-intensive by appointing a task force to define and identify the critical issues affecting the growth and development of those hospice programs. NHO president Carolyn Fitzpatrick said:

> The task force will be asked to identify current and future needs of these hospice programs and to recommend options

available to these programs. The task force will be asked to recommend specific strategies available to volunteer-intensive hospices that will encourage their development. (NHO, 1984).

POTENTIAL CRISES AND CONCERNS

Staff Stress: How to Recognize it and How to Cope

Staff and volunteer stress reactions or "burnout" is a concern of hospice administrators/directors. Once staff stress occurs, it tends to be contagious; therefore, prevention of staff stress is the approach used in hospice programs. The day-in, day-out close contact with dying patients brings the hospice worker into frequent confrontation with his or her own mortality. Staff and volunteer orientation and training programs include personal death and attitude awareness sessions. The nature of hospice care deprives team members of some very effective and comfortable defense mechanisms in dealing with terminal illness and death. Depersonalization, detachment, clear definition of responsibility, and stereotyped responses are the normal and understandable reactions to the threat of a patient's death. However, hospice care is characterized by a high degree of personal attention and involvement, lack of strict role definitions for team members, and an emphasis on flexible and innovative responses to situations (Pelletier, 1977).

Excessive stress leads to a number of undesirable effects, for example, impairment of the team member's capacity to provide excellent patient care, friction between team members, and high turnover rate among hospice personnel. This not only results in considerable dislocation for individual team members but also has an unfavorable impact on the quality of care provided to patients. In order to avoid stress reactions, some hospice programs have a written selection process for team members utilizing individual and/or group interviews which act as guideposts for spotting possible areas of concern regarding staff members. If a potential problem is observed, such as reluctance to care for the dying, negative feelings about death, unresolved grief, emotional instability, or a too recent personal loss, an interview is conducted by the staff support counselor to further analyze the concern. In addition, a group interview may be conducted to observe individual responses within the group process.

Once the staff is selected, proper orientation serves as a tool in preventing staff stress. Mutual sharing and assistance among the members of the hospice team are the most effective weapons in the prevention of harmful team member stress reactions. Educational programs encourage personal growth which, in turn, enhances personal satisfaction. Psychiatric staff are particularly suited to provide support to other team members, and hospice team members are expected to avail themselves of these services freely. Administrators should become concerned about staff members who show little or no interest in support services. Many part-time workers need to work with other types of patients who are curable to reduce stress in caring for the dying. Staff energies can thus be channelled toward other areas of health care, not only toward care for the dying. By use of such "distancing" techniques, staff may act as if they are completely free of hospice responsibilities and concerns at intervals.

The scattered-bed approach does alleviate some of the stress problems related specifically to terminal care. Informal individual counseling is helpful to provide constant reinforcement to those who must frequently deal with the trauma of death and dying. Strong leadership for staff guidance and encouragement is important.

Staff Stress--Symptoms and Coping Mechanisms

A recent analysis in one hospice organization as to sources of staff stress revealed some concerns for administrators. Sources were:

- When diagnosis is unknown to the patient and/or family

- Combining career and erratic hours of hospice work

- Caring for patients who are same age as staff members

- Too many patients at once, especially *very* terminal ones--staff-patient ratio

- "Paperwork"--medical record documentation

- When aggressive therapy is not appropriate--some family physicians tend to continue ordering chemotherapy when no longer effective

- When physician doesn't tell patient true diagnosis--not honest with patient.

Symptoms of stress included irritability, staff reaching out to other caregivers, fatigue, decreased quality of care in that a comprehensive approach is not used with patients such as when personal care is given but not emotional support, frustration, and inability to listen.

Stress management. One major source of staff support in the same hospice is the continuing education component: in this organization, monthly sessions are held which include the important area of stress management. Staff share stories about recent events in their personal or professional lives--both pleasant and unpleasant--and they may exchange ideas for coping. Below is a listing of possible agendas for similar monthly meetings, adopted from one hospice's work in this area:

- Exercises for "values clarification"--individual priorities and how people come to hold certain beliefs and establish certain behavior patterns--and hints on how to prioritize daily activities to reduce personal stress

- Techniques for progressive relaxation

- Discussion of "mirror image stress"-- overidentification of caregiver with the patient/family

- Discussion of personality types attracted to the caregiving professions and ways to prevent overextension of oneself

- Discussion of anger: appropriate and inappropriate; how to express it; when to express it; how to evaluate it; cognitive distortions due to anger; how to handle others' anger; alternate interventions

- Sleep disorders due to grief (a major difficulty for many of the bereaved)

- Summary and discussion of the work of Mary L.S. Vachon: ("Are Your Patients Burning Out?" and "Measurement and Management of Stress in Health Professionals Working with Advanced Cancer Patients").

One additional item worthy of note, which may lead to additional areas for exploration in educational seminars: nursing students who have had the opportunity of working in hospice alongside professional nurses have observed that the hospice caregiver seems more comfortable with silence than nurses they had observed in their previous experience, and they noted that silence itself can be an effective tool at times. Simple touching, the student nurses noted, can be similarly effective. The topics of silence and the "healing touch" may be worth looking into further--not only for the patient/family but for caregivers undergoing stress as well.

Stages and Symptoms. Shubin (1978) describes three progressive stages associated with stress: (1) The first stage is physical and emotional exhaustion, and the beginning of other physical symptoms; (2) the second stage is the development of a negative attitude toward clients, with decreased energy applied to work; (3) the third stage is a feeling of total disgust with work with previous symptoms becoming extreme. By the third stage, burnout may be irreversible.

Physical symptoms of stress include tiredness or exhaustion, headaches, gastrointestinal problems, increased colds, loss of appetite, loss of weight, sleeplessness, and psychosomatic disorders. *Emotional/psychological symptoms* may include general moodiness, detachment, depression, conflict-laden dreams or nightmares, increased irritability, boredom and cynicism, emotional exhaustion, negative feelings towards clients and loss of concern for them, and negative self-image. *Behavioral symptoms* may be increased use of drugs or alcohol, increased absenteeism, impaired performance, lowered productivity, inability to detach from work, increased isolation from others, and increased rigidity in thinking and opposition to new ideas.

Causes of Internal Stress. Overall causes of stress include such internally-generated sources as overextending one's self, not setting limits, working at too fast a pace without sufficient breaks, working under constant pressure, lacking skills in areas necessary to do one's work well, always being a leader, having others depend on you, being an idealist, being a perfectionist, being impatient, wanting to be liked by everyone, not paying attention to one's own needs and wants, not paying attention to diet, exercise, and sleep patterns, not communicating well with others, not sharing intimacies with special others on a regular basis, being overinvolved in a single area of one's life to the exclusion of other areas, feeling overwhelmed by money problems, family problems, or other conflicts, feeling isolated, feeling helpless or powerless, not receiving or accepting positive feedback, and failing to manage stress effectively.

Prevention Strategies. There are a number of useful strategies for preventing or minimizing such stress. Perhaps most important are good communication skills. It is important to know how to be assertive, express anger creatively and effectively, give direct, nonthreatening messages, maintain congruity of verbal, nonverbal, and paralinguistic communications, listen, and maintain a sense of humor. There are numerous body methods of stress management, including massage, progressive relaxation, and breathing exercises. Physical exercise is equally important: jogging, swimming, and walking are popular methods for relaxing the body and thereby reducing stress. Taking care of nutritional needs through proper diet should never be underestimated; neither should the need for physical affection--a well-timed hug can do wonders. There are a number of mind control methods for stress reduction also: meditation, hypnosis/self-hypnosis, visualization techniques, and "practicing" new positive traits and attitudes.

Some of the most important methods of managing stress may be the most obvious. Treat yourself with love and care, engage in pleasurable activities regularly, especially outside of work. Talk to and be with people who care.

In the work arena, there are techniques to minimize stress: take short breaks during the day, improve skills in areas that will help you do your job well, develop realistic expectations, set time limits and priorities, and finally, seek out assistance of others when necessary.

Causes of External Stress and Prevention Strategies. Within the organizational structure itself, there are certain problems that can be a source of staff stress. Among them are a high client-to-staff ratio, a lack of positive feedback, a lack of adequate supervision, no opportunity for upward mobility, and a lack of staff involvement in policy making. A hospice administrator, therefore, should try to maintain a reasonable client-to-staff ratio, provide opportunities for upward--or even lateral--mobility, encourage staff participation in policy making, sanction a number of sick days as "mental health" days, encourage staff to take vacations, develop on-the-job support systems, and educate staff about burnout syndrome (Galinsky, 1982; Vachon, 1982).

In their preliminary studies on staff stress, Vachon *et al.* found that nurses in an active treatment cancer hospital were found to focus on problems with dying patients as a displacement for their feelings of inadequacy in stressful conditions. Major problems with various aspects of the work situation and with staff communications were cited just as often as problems in watching people suffer and die. This finding maximizes the role of the administration and the importance of effective organization and management within an organization.

Stress among physicians was also observed in the study. The most valuable service to physicians is an effective referral system that deals with psychosocial aspects of patient and families, a weak area for physicians generally. Again, educational programs are indicated which deal with the psychosocial aspects of cancer (Vachon, *et al.*, 1978).

Hospice administrators must be able to identify symptoms of stress and readily adapt strategies for overcoming ongoing stressful situations.

Medical Ethics

Medical ethics in relation to ordinary versus extraordinary means of caring for the dying is an unavoidable question, and one that goes to the heart of the morality of caring for the dying. This concern must be addressed in the written policies and procedures of hospice programs as well as by an established philosophy evidenced in hospice policy manuals, that is, palliative care as a purpose for the hospice program of care.

Acceptance of hospice care is not an appropriate coping mechanism for all individuals. Nonacceptance by the patient can be expected to occur at times. A review of potential referrals during hospice site visits showed evidence that some patients were not admitted because they did not accept the hospice program as discussed in Chapter I.

The question of pain control in hospice care is crucial. Hospice philosophy dictates that pain medication be given on a regular basis around the clock and not on a whenever-necessary routine. The degree to which this standard is upheld seems to depend on the physician rather than the type of hospice. Education of physicians and nurses as to hospice pain control practice is necessary if hospice criterion is to be met.

The single most important factor in determining the success of a hospice program is the quality of the people who work in it. Some staff truly derive authentic personal satisfaction from hospice involvement because of their discontent with the health care delivery system. Still, various "staffing problems" and conflicts arise periodically. Staff members can exhibit sensitivity and dedication, but their motivation may be for self and not for helping others. The growth of a hospice program may also become a problem to some staff because of their own limitations and deficiencies resulting from lack of formal education and disinterest in or inability to participate in continuing education mechanisms. Besides being caring and sensitive, individuals may need other technical skills to succeed in a hospice environment.

Staff involvement may be less than ideal in terms of their own possibly skewed goals and dissatisfaction in working with the dying patient. Many people who want to work with hospice have a sense of calling, an almost missionary zeal which hospice may not be able to satisfy. Individuals without supportive relationships may be unable to obtain the personal support necessary to offset the emotionally draining nature of hospice work. Staff selection should be done in a manner to screen those individuals not right for hospice caregiving. A prospective staff member's social support system should be carefully assessed (Vachon, 1983). A sixty-day probationary period with extensive orientation and intensive training should allow the supervisor time to observe, monitor, and evaluate each new staff member on a one-to-one basis.

If the individual isn't functioning at an expected level of expertise within sixty days, he or she is not an appropriate hospice staff member. Many nurses, for example, enter the profession to work at the bedside with patients only to find that their role has changed. In the conventional setting, this individual may find him/herself spending most of the time away from the bedside, writing medical records, making rounds with physicians, and in a supervisory role. He or she comes to hospice in order to give personal care again such as bed baths and treatments, but may not really want to care for dying patients who require special emotional care as well. Hospice care may therefore become a conflict rather than a satisfying experience.

Special Needs of Children and Young Adults

Children with Cancer. Hospice programs throughout the United States need to focus attention on the needs of the dying child and their loved ones. The American Academy of Pediatrics supports hospice care for children. Their approval was strengthened by a report from Dr. Robert Milch, associate surgery professor at State University of New York at Buffalo. Milch (1984) states that "hospice is the most humane way to care for patients in the last stages of life, patients who are terminally ill. Hospice isn't just for adults."

A child needs the emotional support, understanding, and physical security provided by his or her parents, brothers, sisters, and significant others as well as proper medical attention. It is better for a child to die in a homelike environment. Therefore, the emphasis is now on treating the child with cancer at home or as close to home as possible in order to limit disruption of normal family activity. However, some parents still find comfort in continued hospitalization in order to feel they are doing everything possible for the sick child.

The Ronald McDonald House, a concept which began in Philadelphia in 1974, is a place where families can stay when medical care has to be provided a distance from their home. The concept was supported by the fund-raising efforts of McDonald's restaurants. A Ronald McDonald House is only a temporary residence for families. It is not a medical treatment facility, a hospice, hotel, motel or psychotherapy unit. However, families do draw additional strength and find stability there when a child is seriously ill. By late 1985, there were 89 Ronald McDonald Houses operating internationally: 77 in the United States, 10 in Canada, one in Sydney, Australia, and one in the Netherlands. The network is expanding rapidly; 27 houses are under renovation or construction and 45 additional sites are under consideration (Jones, 1985).

Children do fear separation from parents before death. Admission to a hospital increases this fear. Therefore, a specialized hospice unit which understands the special needs of children and young adults is appropriate. The nation's first full-service children's hospice with ten inpatient beds and a capacity for fifty children, age sixteen and younger, in the home care program opened at St. Mary's Hospital for Children in Bayside, New York. Stewart (1984) describes the unit as an environment with brightly painted walls and no nurse's station. Children wear their own clothes, not hospital pajamas and there is a room full of arcade video games. Children are there for changes of pain medication and symptom control.

Children possess a life-oriented attitude as they go about their daily activities. There is little evidence that they fear death. It is most important, however, to help a dying child talk about his illness. He or she may want to "open up"; therefore, the hospice team member must be extremely alert to cues for discussion. Spiritually, a child is comforted by the belief he will go to heaven when he dies. Children with cancer often plan for the future; they may believe they will live forever and that they have control and power over everything.

Parents of a dying child who also have other children at home often feel guilty for neglecting the other children in the family. Hospice caregivers need to assist parents in learning to acknowledge this guilt and gain a balanced perspective on it. Support groups should be formed for the family. One such organization exists throughout the nation: Candlelighters. This group helps families deal with psychological problems and monitors the quality of care for childhood cancer patients (Clifford, 1979).

Denial in children should not be considered only negative; it may be healthy. The reality of death must be recognized, but both parents and child should lead as normal a life as possible. Parents should not sit around constantly depressed and crying. They, too, need a positive life-oriented attitude.

Children of Cancer Patients. On the other side of the coin, children of dying patients also have special needs. Children and teenagers have special problems when cancer or any life-threatening illness occurs in their families. The hospice care team must encourage families to take time to listen to their child's feelings and spend time with them. Make Today Count, Inc. has information and helpful suggestions for families with children such as when and how much to tell the children.*

A new Arts-in-Hospice program has been developed at Hospice of the Good Shepherd, Inc., Waban, Maine. Hospice staff in this program are concerned with the creative as well as the physical needs of their patients. Ginny Foy, Hospice Arts Coordinator, explains: "Art allows patients an opportunity to regain a feeling of self-esteem and a sense of control over their lives. It allows families to share in a creative experience bringing family members together." Creative arts play a role with terminally ill patients, their families and the hospice teams that serve them. The evolution of a Kids' Arts program has been most effective in children of hospice becoming creative survivors (Foy, 1984).

Ever-Kare, Inc. provides guidelines on explaining death to children in their publication *Bereavement Counseling: Your Start To A New Life*, as follows:

1. Death education should be a part of the children's normal education.

2. Death should be explained to children in a comfortable atmosphere.

3. Death should be explained to children by someone whom they trust.

4. Children should know that they will be taken care of.

5. Children should know that the dead person will not return.

6. Children should not be afraid to express their emotions.

7. The children should know that the adults will also be grieving. (Van Fleteren, 1983)

Parental debate over when and how much to tell the children, disruption of normal household activity, physical changes in a loved one all add to the tension of a family already burdened. Parent and Child Guidance Center in Pittsburgh, PA, a group that works with children of chronically ill parents, offers the following helpful suggestions for families:

- Take time to listen to the child's feelings. Accept them for they are real. Don't try to talk him or her out of them or deny them.

- Provide honest information at the child's level without frightening him or her. Answer all the questions. Fantasies can be scarier than reality.

- Understand that the child may need to ask the same questions over and over again.

---

*Information available through Make Today Count, Inc., P.O. Box 222, Osage Beach, MO 65065.

- Recognize that the child may have worries about abandonment. "Will my other parent get sick, too?" "Who will take care of me?" Reassure the child that the healthy parent can and will provide care.

- Prepare the child about the effects of different medications on mom or dad.

- Older children can certainly help with the younger children but care should be taken that they are not given more responsibility than they are ready for or put in the role of a substitute parent.

- Find time to spend with the children. The ill parent will have some good hours. The healthy parent can set some priorities. Does it matter if the laundry doesn't get done today?

- Avoid making children feel guilty.

- Reassure children, younger ones especially, who get sick that they are not in danger of becoming as sick as mom or dad.

- Recognize the importance of play as a way for a young child to work on his feelings. Support it without interference.

- If the child has a creative and understanding teacher who knows the situation, the teacher may be able to devise some ways in the classroom to enable the child's classmates to understand and make him feel less isolated (Kelly, 1985).

More and more hospice programs are becoming aware of the special needs of children in hospice both as dying patients themselves and as survivors. As specialized needs become more complex, hospice consultants and caregiving professionals are developing innovative programs and disseminating educational materials for professional use.

Other Possible Areas for Concern

Lack of evaluation of hospice programs in the hospital model was evidenced by the findings of the author's research in Chapter 8. This is identified as critical by this author as program evaluation is required for most funding sources. Furthermore, the quality of care being provided in the hospice program is determined formally through evaluation. The effectiveness of patient care, staff function, and the impact of the program on the medical community, the institutional community, and the general public should be covered in the evaluation. Finally, a comprehensive and thorough evaluation requires a well-planned program (Torrens, 1985).

Future crises may involve legal, ethical, and political aspects in the delivery of hospice care.   In hospice models, an intensive analysis of the internal dynamics is complex. Future problems in delivery of hospice care are likely to involve interorganizational conflicts. The attitude of the hospice staff greatly affects its quality. Derisiveness about what can and should be done for terminally ill patients and their families can only impede hospice progress and be counter-productive to quality hospice care. For a team of professionals to blend their skills in a responsible way--especially when most members have been accustomed in their work setting to a traditional hierarchy--a substantial social adjustment is required. This is unexplored territory in health care employment; mutual obligation, mutual sharing of responsibility, and a sense of shared ethical obligations; each member of the hospice team must feel responsible for what his or her colleagues do or fail to do. Clinical practitioners who have heard and continue to hear the lonely voices of patients and families should remain in the forefront of all new efforts. Their close connection with patients must be the strength behind the principles of hospice care.

The organizational process and the struggle for control can endanger the democratic quality of the movement and influence the human services it gives. The sense of a total community needs to survive the technological innovations of institutions. Safeguards need to be placed on administrative practices to ensure a continuing commitment to hospice principles.   Despite all of the official administrative support possible, the hospice team members must realize they are in unfriendly territory. People are political and maneuver for power and money; the hospice staff members may have to struggle in order to establish their turf.

The hospice movement, without attempting to resolve euthanasia issues, seems to help strengthen patients' will to live by providing quality of life in the remaining days. The public needs to be educated about the hospice philosophy of care.

Continued reliance on the use of volunteers for direct services may present future problems if hospice programs do not plan ahead for provision of ongoing services. Recruitment of volunteers is vitally important to the program. In an era of generally declining volunteerism, most hospice programs have found that volunteers are available. The work is interesting and rewarding, but even more appealing to many volunteers is the willingness of hospice programs to give them responsibility. For this reason, superlative programs must be designed for volunteers to improve and develop specific skills and sensitivities in such areas as individual and group dynamics, supportive counseling, and listening skills.

THE FUTURE OF HOSPICE

In researching written material on the future of the hospice movement, this writer was impressed with the variety and shades of opinion among accredited authors, medical professionals, clergy, and laypersons intimately associated with hospice as expressed in books, manuals, essays, medical journals, magazine articles, and so on. These opinions varied in tone: the early articles in the late 1960s tended to be tinged with the heightened enthusiasm of the idealist; in the mid-1970s a more cautious optimism was expressed. Finally, a more realistic assessment of the hospice movement developed; some authors expressed a slightly more pessimistic approach about how soon the ideals of the original hospice concept of the late 1960s might be achieved.

The recent rash of "realists" took into consideration the other concerns that currently exist nationally. Uncertain economic conditions and skyrocketing inflation have contributed to the ever-increasing costs of health care services. The Reagan Administration cut the budgets of many government grants and subsidies. At this time, therefore, the future of hospice funding is uncertain. Some writers forecast that while hospice will indubitably continue as a part of the American health care scene, it seems destined, apparently, to assume a more standardized role than exists today. Confusion exists as to the adoption of the "ideal" hospice model. The trend, it appears, is towards the hospice home care model, but adequate funding is the crux of the problem. However, even though government grants may dwindle, the hospice movement is already vitally rooted in the American health care scene.

Based on my own summary research findings, a community-based hospice (such as a certified home health agency in conjunction with a hospital-based inpatient unit administered by the community hospice team) is the suggested model for the future. The community-based model of hospice care serves not only as a direct provider but as a coordinator of those health care services presently existing in the community. Community health care services are not intended to be duplicated by hospice, rather they are meant to be utilized and integrated into their movement and philosophy. This is, unquestionably, a positive step towards integrating hospice care into an already existing health care system in the community. Planning for new hospice programs must be coordinated with the regional Health Systems Agency (HSA).

Licensing and Duplication of Services

P.L. 93-641 charges the states with reducing health expenditures by eliminating unnecessary or duplicative services. State Health Planning and Development Agencies (SHPDAs) must assess the health care needs of their own state's population with the advice of the State Health Coordinating Council (SHCC). Theoretically, then, every health care provider must document the need for the new service and demonstrate to both the SHPDA and the SHCC that it conforms to the state plan. If the provider successfully proves the necessity of the service, a certificate is granted where appropriate.

The impact of a hospice program upon similar services is perhaps the key to determining duplication of service. If other hospices exist in the applicant's community, a rather clear-cut question arises of the necessity for an additional program. Hospice proponents need to explain the need for a hospice facility in a community full of surplus hospital beds or for hospice home care in an area with established home care agencies. As a matter of policy, both hospitals and nursing services may oppose the hospice applicant's entry into the field. Each has the right to submit written or verbal testimony before the SHPDA and SHCC. Either may claim that the existence of a hospice merely duplicates the services they offer and would lead to further surpluses and, ultimately, higher costs to consumers. In a few states, opponents have successfully blocked the hospice's attempt to secure a certificate of need and these denials were reversed on appeal only after planning authorities were convinced of the clear distinction between hospice care and other home care or hospitalization. State licensure laws vary. In Pennsylvania there is no licensure for home health agencies or hospices.

Currently, about 95 percent of all hospice programs providing nursing care operate under traditional licensure models that were developed for acute, skilled-nursing facilities or home care. Traditional licensure coverage for a hospice program is easy to arrange; institution-based hospices are already covered by their parent organizations. Separate state licensure, therefore, should not be an immediate concern for most beginning hospice programs. In considering licensure/certification for home care, a hospice can either apply for licensure/certification itself or work out a relationship with an agency already having licensure. A hospice applying for its own licensure, however, must consider the effort and cost of setting up a billing mechanism and the stress and vulnerability inherent in periodic evaluations, record reviews, and regulation (Ames, 1980). Hopefully, this approach will remove the abrasiveness and antagonism that has confronted hospice in some communities. Needless to say, the community-based model still embodies and best retains the overall hospice philosophy.

In the future, conceivably, hospital-based hospices will eventually merge with home care in order to provide hospice services to those who require hospitalization. Conversely, the home care models may ultimately merge with hospital-based models, or they may contract separately for inpatient beds. This, for example, is the current arrangement between some West coast functioning hospices (Worby, Blackman, and Schneider, 1978).

There are philosophical, organizational, and financial reasons for promoting the growth of hospital-based units with home care. Experience coupled with research confirms that the hospital-based hospice is not only a possible but also a desirable alternative approach. Optimal care of the terminally ill lies in programs that are truly comprehensive in that they offer continuity of care as the patient shifts from one level to another. Hospice programs should be organized so as to enable the application of hospice principles and practice across the entire spectrum. It will be imperative for hospital-based programs to offer care not only in the hospital but in the home, as well as to patients who require institutionalization in an intermediate-care facility. Any freestanding units will need to develop formalized arrangements that will permit the preservation of continuity of care when patients require hospital care. Relationships will need to be cultivated that permit easy transition between levels of care for a continuum of services. Programs that begin with a home care base will need to find the means whereby patients can receive care in skilled and intermediate care facilities and in hospitals without loss of continuity of care. One of the strengths of hospice thus far has been its diversity of form and style. Successful hospice programs have adapted to local needs. Whatever the origin and whatever the center for operations, the ultimate aim of hospice programs is going to be the provision of comprehensive care. Otherwise, hospice will run the danger of perpetuating the kind of fragmentation which has plagued the conventional approach which it seeks to replace.

Education for the Future

The inclusion of courses dealing with dying in the curriculum of universities and high schools is needed. The lack of public and professional insight into the dying process is evidenced because of the intensive counseling required by the specialized hospice team. The study of death and dying, or thanatology, must begin in the primary schools. Modern psychologists agree that the minds of young students are most impressionable at this stage of growth and development. My own experience in teaching the hospice concept to junior and senior high school students validates this observation. I have found the students to be especially receptive and responsive. During these sessions on death and dying, some students identify well, particularly those who have lost loved ones. They develop an understanding that grief is a normal process. This indicates that death and dying education may begin in the home where parents probably have the most profound influence on the minds of their young children. The progressive school administrator may consider this subject of thanatology a challenge and initiate these classes in their own districts to further benefit the students. No better background of the knowledge of hospice care could benefit the hospice movement more.

Resources for Future Funding

The limited reimbursement for hospice services such as twenty-four-hour supportive and nonskilled care and death and dying and bereavement counseling becomes an ongoing problem for hospice administrators. Hospice educators must continue to stress among both legislators and the public alike, the difference between "hospice" care principles and traditional care. Furthermore, everyone must be made to understand that "hospice" is a program providing a continuum of care for patients and families, not necessarily a specific place.

States should develop guidelines for assuring the public that the highest quality of care will be rendered to the terminally ill. However, restraint should be exercised in promulgating regulations for the control of hospice. Excessive, demanding, and troublesome government regulations with limited reimbursement has exerted an inhibitory effect on developing hospices instead of encouraging the growth of this new discipline. State governments should begin to offer assistance rather than oppose the implementation of hospice care facilities at a time when specialized care to the chronically and terminally ill patient and family is so critical.

Unfortunately, the traditional profit-oriented principles of corporations and the limited government support at this juncture leaves the hospice movement without any sound base of adequate funding. It has been stated by hospice administrators that the lack of money and public understanding is the crux of the whole problem confronting the hospice movement today.

As the hospice movement continues to expand, those concerned with it must find a way to strike a balance between principles and ideals on the one hand and political and economic realities on the other (Wald, Foster, and Wald, 1980).

Here again, hospice services are implemented and programs developed based on the availability of funding. Insurance companies must continue to reexamine their policy of providing benefits for medical services that treat curative disease only. Society is slowly realizing that it would be far more beneficial for these companies to treat the patient as a whole, whether he remains in the hospital or at home. Cohen (1979) advocates that the holistic approach rather than the curing of disease must be emphasized in the future. Reimbursement is also needed for bereavement counseling.

Hospice program development continues to be considerably ahead of any significant advancements in the preparedness of health insurers and rulemakers to adequately reimburse or mandate licensure for hospice type care (Armado, 1980). The ongoing challenge is to convert the ideals of hospice into practical terms which consider the realities of quality control and reimbursement while still remaining faithful to those original ideals. Hospice is a response to certain needs of the terminally ill that are not being met by standard health care programs (Hadlock, 1980).

Valid statistical measures, in-depth program evaluation, and accurate financial analyses will only enhance reimbursement prospects for hospice care. While it is encouraging to find evidence of cost efficiency, it is of little value unless the program meets its objectives and standards.

The Reagan Administration's cutback policies reducing funds available to Medicare and other medical assistance programs are significant to hospice administrators. Therefore, the public must be made increasingly aware of the hospice movement in order to promote private contributions and public funding drives nationally. This may compensate in part for the projected deficit in necessary operational costs.

Clarification of cost and reimbursement issues must be concomitant with resolution of the organizational problems in hospice care. Decisions in these areas are matters of public policy and will have to be addressed in this fashion. The health consumer will have to determine for what he or she wishes to pay.

The role of hospice leaders is to inform the public of what is available, so that consumers can make intelligent choices (Zimmerman, 1981).

REMAINING QUESTIONS

There are a number of questions which still remain. Is care of the terminally ill important, or should our financial resources be directed primarily at curative and rehabilitative medicine? If we are to reimburse for terminal care, what services should be reimbursed and at what price? Should bereavement counseling be reimbursable? At what levels should services be reimbursed? What sort of organizational format should we require of those providing terminal care in order to be eligible for reimbursement? What comprehensive coverage can be provided for the delivery of care at home? Should eligibility criteria be expanded in hospice programs to allow the application of the hospice concept to those with lingering terminal illnesses? Should hospice program evaluation include patient care provided by hospital staff not employed by hospice (when a patient is hospitalized in a facility without a hospice unit)? Should reimbursement include art and music therapy? Should pastoral counseling be a reimbursable service? Should hospice become an alternate delivery system along with preferred provider organizations and health maintenance organizations?

It is the legislatures and insurance companies, presumably on the basis of public preference, which establish the services that will be reimbursed and the formulae for that reimbursement. They need to be particularly well-informed about issues relating to the care of the terminally ill (Zimmerman, 1981). The current $6,500 cap on total benefits to a hospice patient combined with low rates set by HHS and a highly structured benefit package has kept many hospices from participating in the Hospice Medicare program. The National Hospice Reimbursement Act of 1982 as discussed earlier is headed for a sunset in 1986. Testimonies must continue to save the Medicare Hospice Benefit from certain failure. Even though Congress responded to months of intensive effort and passed legislation to increase the reimbursement level for routine hospice care to $53.17 per day, up from $46.25, NHO has found the cost of providing routine home care to be $70.47. The legislation, effective October 1, 1984, requires that the Secretary of Department of HHS review the adequacy of all hospice rates not less than annually.

As hospice systems evolve and matters of reimbursement are settled, the role of volunteers in hospice care will require close scrutiny and careful thought. The contribution of volunteers to the success of hospices has been enormous based on the findings of the author's research, that is, results of medical record audit, questionnaire responses, and interviews with directors who discussed the need to involve volunteers in bereavement programs. This contribution has, in part, been through the provision of services which have made the volunteers effective extenders of the professionals in the health care system. This has had a tremendous financial impact. In some instances, it has made hospice care possible, for it is only in this way that the high level of personal attention which hospice care requires could be provided. But, in addition, volunteers have contributed in another important respect; they have brought values and viewpoints that have refreshed and strengthened hospice programs (Zimmerman, 1981).

To the extent that hospice care becomes more integrated into the health care system, as accreditation of hospice programs expand and as reimbursement for hospice care becomes more widely available, there is clearly a threat to volunteer involvement in hospice. The necessary steps must be taken to preserve volunteer participation above and beyond legislative mandates.

As hospice moves closer to universal licensure and ongoing reimbursement, it also moves closer to full integration into the health care system. This raises certain questions; Do volunteers who fit into a changing system risk losing the unique role they have filled in the pioneering phase of hospice development? The hospice volunteer is as specialized as any other member of the hospice caring team. The careful selection process and extensive training utilized by most programs emphasize this specialization. The various roles fulfilled by hospice volunteers is more extensively involved in the direct provision of patient care than it is in other health care settings, a requirement for participation in the hospice Medicare Benefit Program discussed earlier. Medical record audit of the types of volunteer services showed that 42 percent of the patients received companion services, 19 percent received respite care, 10 percent received transportation, 4 percent homemaking, 4 percent errands, and 5 percent received direct patient care from volunteers. Volunteers from the hospitals studied providing services to other than the hospice program do not provide any direct services to patients within those institutions. What seems to set hospice volunteers apart, according to Lorenz (1980), is more qualitative than quantitative. As members of the provider team, volunteers are expected to not only supplement staff functions, but also to give of themselves as individuals, to become personally involved, yet to remain objective in the care they provide. The perceptions and opinions of hospice volunteers as team members are respected; this creates an unusual circumstance within the health field. Care must be taken not to allow the role of volunteers to become blurred or lost.

As new programs develop and expand or are incorporated into existing structures and as new challenges and concerns are confronted, continued effort is needed to maintain this carefully developed and cultivated caregiving role. The role of the volunteers is expanding in hospice programs. Hospice care should be viewed as part of a continuum of care--an option that should be available to patients and their families as a matter of choice. Toward this end, new and flexible sources of public and private financing are needed, and multiple points of entry to the care system must be established. Home care and other kinds of extrainstitutional care, treatment, and services, furnished by an interdisciplinary team of professionals and volunteers on bases that are likely to be nontraditional, must be made available. New concepts of choice on the part of patients and families must be recognized. The quality of life, not merely its prolongation, should be of central concern. Accordingly, a wide range of drugs, medications, and other techniques to alleviate physical and emotional pain should be more readily utilized.

This discussion would not be complete without some emphasis on the role of the various members of the hospice team beyond the traditional nurse and doctor team. The use of the interdisciplinary team is critical in providing quality of care--an area which became an emphasis as a result of the author's research. From medical record audit, a relationship is observed between lack of a formal educational program and limited use of the interdisciplinary team.

The recruitment, selection, training, and integration of the interdisciplinary team is the central theme of hospice. This requires a major administrative and supervisory effort. *Professional direction and implementation of the team approach, augmented by volunteers, is the most important criterion for the welfare of the terminally ill patient/family.*

Effective work with dying patients and their families requires special knowledge, skills, and sensitivity. Moreover, the emotional demands of hospice care on both professional and lay staff and volunteers are substantial. A need for ongoing staff education is evidenced. To be sure, in the health care industry today, all health care professionals would benefit from a hospice institute, an educational institution providing the training and skills of sensitive care. Staff members themselves recognized the need for continued classes/conferences in order to upgrade the quality of care they provide to terminally ill patients. Training opportunities must be expanded, and training methods must constantly be reassessed and reevaluated. Regular conferences utilizing cases available in the program are an extremely valuable teaching tool. This needs to be supplemented by periodic topic-oriented instruction covering such matters as the control of specific symptoms, techniques of dealing with grief reactions, and new methods in tumor control. Staff members should visit other hospice programs and meetings to gain additional knowledge of hospice care and skills to prevent stress reactions and/or burnout. Maintaining an updated indexed list of recommended readings can be very helpful and must be made available within the hospice library. The need for respite, either as part of in-service staff development programs or in conjunction with other training activities, must be recognized and provided.

The role of professional social work must be viewed as integral to hospice care. The goal of social work service is to help the patient and family deal with the personal and social problems of illness, disability, and impending death. The social worker, through a psycho-social assessment, addresses the problems, needs, and capacities of the patient and his or her family and brings to the hospice team a special knowledge of community resources. He or she is involved in provision of supportive and therapeutic counseling, care planning, direct assistance to the patient and his or her family, and in the bereavement counseling. In many ways, the hospice is the embodiment of social work values, principles, and practice. Social work has a long history of direct service to dying patients and their families. This strengthens the role of the social worker as a member of the hospice care team in dealing with social and emotional aspects of care. Social workers are familiar with the crisis of fatal illness and its grave impact on personal resources and the very nature and continuity of family life. Among the interventions of social work are the use of helping skills to mediate the struggle of the dying patient and the family to cope, to communicate, and to resolve the inner and outer forces bearing down during this life crisis (Foster, 1979). Moreover, the special knowledge and skills of professional social workers in providing direct services, in administration, in volunteer and staff training, in working with patients, families and community, in case management, and in utilizing and coordinating community resources and volunteers are indispensible to an effective hospice program. In many ways, social workers become attitude adjustment therapists. All hospice patients and families are seen by a social worker so that the social, emotional, environmental, and financial impact of the terminal illness may be evaluated.

The variations in the administration of the bereavement counseling programs both among and within hospice programs demonstrate the necessity for further development of a unique program that provides a continuum of supportive and therapeutic services for the family including formal and informal individual, family, and group treatment modalities. These should be employed as needed to support the patient's family for at least one year to eighteen months following death since periods around anniversaries, birthdays, and holidays are difficult during this time.

The whole population benefits from humanistic health care practices. Because the patient and family are an interacting system, holistic practice dictates that they be treated as a single unit. Each member affects the other, as does any change in family status. Family members become a component part of the hospice team. Although an interdisciplinary approach is fundamental to hospice care, to reach its full potential a hospice program must, in the final analysis, be a medical program. Many health care professionals and administrators believe that the medical model is necessary in health care today. All reimbursement conditions require medical certification. Physician participants must indeed be prepared to function as team members and to share responsibility. To attempt to operate a hospice care program without active physician involvement results in either failure or the development of a program which exists outside of the conventional care system, leading to future fragmentation and inevitably, poorer patient care. All hospice models require a medical director on staff who acts as staff physician or consultant.

Finally, according to national standards, hospice programs--regardless of the model of care--should develop resources to meet the moral and religious needs of patients and their families. Pastoral care services must be further developed to both respect and serve the spiritual needs of hospice patients/families who desire pastoral care services. This includes educational programs for hospice staff *and* community clergy. The pastoral counselor becomes an important member of the interdisciplinary hospice care team in order to meet physical, emotional, spiritual, and social needs of the hospice patient and family.

AIDS--A NEW DIAGNOSIS IN HOSPICE PROGRAMS

Acquired immunodeficiency syndrome, or AIDS, is a new illness that involves a complexity of health problems in which patients develop a severe loss of their natural immunity against disease. It is characterized by immunodeficiency, opportunistic infections, and unusual malignant diseases. Kaposi's sarcoma has developed in approximately one-third of patients with AIDS (Gilmore, *et al.*, 1983).

As of April 29, 1985, 9,953 patients with AIDS have been reported to the Centers for Disease Control in Atlanta, Georgia. Of these, 4,906 or 49% have died (CDC, 1985). Most of the surviving AIDS patients are expected to die from an opportunistic disease eventually (Popkin, 1983). Dr. Henry Masur of the National Institutes of Health notes that none of the victims he has studied has lived more than 18 months. "Once they develop a severe case of the disease, I suspect they all die," he says (Clark, *et al.*, 1983). Patients who get over one infection often contract another, and that is why their prospects for recovery are so poor. Individuals at risk include male homosexuals (71%), I.V. drug abusers (17%), Haitian refugees (5%), and hemophiliacs and recipients of blood products (6%) (Jemison-Smith, *et al.*, 1983).

Geographical distribution is pertinent to hospice administrators throughout the country since nearly half of the reported cases have been from New York and approximately 20% from California. Cases have also been reported from more than 30 states. Because of increased mobility of individuals today, as well as the stigma of the disease itself, hospice programs need to be prepared for caring for AIDS patients and their families. Experiences of this author have revealed that often AIDS patients who may have lived temporarily in the metropolitan areas return to the homes of their parents and loved ones in smaller communities for care.

Hospice caregivers have a heightened sense of compassion toward dying patients which is naturally crucial in working with AIDS patients. Equally important is aggressive patient advocacy. A true hospice professional cares, regardless of personal feelings. One senior staff nurse in a medical unit found physician and staff education to be critical in ensuring that caregivers understand that AIDS patients/families also need humane and tolerant treatment and to approach their care fearlessly. Staff education included seminars on AIDS with speakers from the Centers for Disease Control and orientation classes to all new staff members (Moran, 1985). Indeed, all hospice libraries should include the latest information on AIDS.

Patient education programs help reduce feelings of isolation and degradation. In explaining isolation rationales, focus should be on the source of infection, not on the patient or overall disease. The use of special procedures for infection control must be carefully interpreted to patients.

The hospice care team must be especially concerned with infection control when managing AIDS patients because of the possibility of carrying infection to AIDS patients who are themselves immunocompromised. Strict regard for precautions will also protect the caregivers themselves and other patients with compromised immune systems from possible infection by AIDS patients. Specific precautionary techniques must be developed by all hospice programs specific to the care of AIDS patients.

Key points to include in isolation techniques when caring for AIDS patients are:

- Gloves whenever you must come in direct contact with the patient's body fluids, secretions, or excretions. Wash your hands after removing the gloves and before leaving the patient's room.

- Gown only when the patient has copious secretions or excretions.

- Mask only when performing a procedure in which secretions or excretions may splatter inadvertently (Popkin, 1983).

Changes in a patient's social and psychological status can present the most challenging problems. Besides enduring physical isolation with numerous precautions, AIDS victims must contend with societal attitudes toward homosexuals. Symptoms such as fatigue and a diagnosis of cancer lower their self-esteem. As a result, AIDS patients experience a change in body image and change in their ability to fulfill their sexual needs (SoRelle, 1985). Sensitive and well-informed hospice care team members who are specially trained in all these areas are critical to the quality of care to AIDS patients.

The implications for the hospice care team are many. A diagnosis of cancer or some other terminal disease is heavy enough. But add to that the fact that the patients are young, most of them in their 20's and early 30's--then tell them their disease that may kill them while they are young is due to their sexual behavior-- then tell them it is due to their gay sexual behavior--and then tell them it may be infectious. This creates many unpleasant feelings--guilt, anger, remorse, depression, despair, fear of desertion (Henig, 1983).

Fortunately, homosexual communities in major cities have set up support groups that provide information and guidance for victims and raise money for research.

Certainly all aspects of hospice care, coupled with a sensitive interdisciplinary team and a formal and informal staff support system, are imperative in the care of patients who are diagnosed with AIDS. As more information about the disease is learned, isolation techniques have become more rigid. Quality nursing care can be provided by isolating the disease through special techniques without necessarily isolating the patient emotionally. A caring, compassionate, and fearless approach to care is essential to both the patient and family as we await breakthroughs in the treatment of AIDS.

REFERENCES

Ames, Richard P. (1980). Starting a Hospice Requires Tenacity, High Standards. *Hospital Progress* 61:56-59.

Armado, Anthony J. (1980). *Chairman of the NHO Committee on Reimbursement and Licensure, Annual Report to the Membership of the National Hospice Organization.* McLean, VA: National Hospice Organization.

Centers for Disease Control. (1985). Telephone conference with author, May 6th.

Clark, Matt, Mariana Gasnell, and Deborah Witherspoon. (1982). AIDS: A Lethal Mystery Story. *Newsweek* (Dec. 27): 63-64.

Clifford, Anne. (1979). Children With Cancer Life-Oriented. *Scranton Times* (PA). April 20th.

Cohen, Kenneth P. (1979). *Hospice Prescription for Terminal Care.* Rockville, MD: Aspen Systems Corporation.

Foster, Zelda. (1979). Standards for Hospice Care: Assumptions and Principles. *Health and Social Work* 4(1):118-128.

Foy, Virginia L. (1984). Workshop on "Arts-In-Hospice" at the National Hospice Organization Annual Meeting, Hartford, CT, November.

Galinsky, Ronald C. (1982). Staff Stress and Career Burnout. Chapter in *Care of the Terminally Ill Manual: Guide to Professional Training.* Published jointly by Riverside Hospice, Boonton, NJ, and the Office of Consumer Health Education, Department of Community Environment and Medicine, Rutgers Medical School, Piscataway, NJ.

Gilmore, N. J., R. Beaulier, M. Steben, and M. Laverdiere. (1983). AIDS: Acquired Immunodeficiency Syndrome. *Canadian Medical Association Journal* 128(6): 1281-1284.

Hadlock, Daniel. (1980). President's Message. NHO Membership Newsletter, McLean, VA.

Halper, Thomas. (1979). On Death, Dying and Terminality: Today, Yesterday and Tomorrow. *Journal of Health Politics, Policy and Law* 4(1):11-29.

Health Resources Publishing. (1984). *Hospice Letter.* 6(6): entire issue.

Henig, Robin Marantz. (1983). AIDS: A New Disease's Deadly Odyssey. *New York Times Magazine* (Feb. 6): 28-44.

Jemison-Smith, Pearl, and Patricia Hamm. (1983). Infection Control Update! *Critical Care Update* 3:30-31.

Jones, Bud. (National Ronald McDonald House Coordinator). (1985). Telephone interview, October 4th.

Kelly, Orville. (1985). Patient's Children Have Special Needs. Prepared by Springfield, MO chapter of Make Today Count, Inc., from *Make Today Count* and *Until Tomorrow Comes.*

Lorenz, Lois. (1980). The Hospice Volunteer, Unique Among Volunteers. *Hospice Forum* 1(3):1-2.

Magno, Josefina B., M.D. (Executive Director of NHO). (1981). Letter To Membership. August 18th.

Miccio, Betty Lou. (1984). A Practical Approach To Quality Assurance for Hospice. *The American Journal of Hospice Care* 1(3):14-15.

Milch, Robert, M.D. (1984). Quoted in article, Hospice Care Turns Attention to Children. *USA Today,* (October 31):section D, 5-6.

Moran, Libby. (1985). The Most Difficult Person I've Ever Worked with--Dr. Cornwall was Obsessed with A.I.D.S. *Nursing Life* 1:30-31.

Mount, Balfour M. (1984). Hospice Expert Sees Doctors' Participation as Key to Programs. *Outreach* 5(5):5.

National Association of Social Work. New York Chapter. (1981). *Proposed Policy Statement: Hospice Care.* New York.

National Hospice Organization. (1984). *Hospice News* 2(5):1.

_____. (1984). New Study Shows Hospice Improves Hospital Care. *Hospice News* 2(5):4.

Pelletier, K. (1977). *Mind As Healer, Mind As Slayer.* New York: Dell.

Popkin, Barbara. (1983). Nursing Ground Rounds--Caring for the AIDS Patient--Fearlessly. *Nursing 83* 13(9): 50-55.

Seguine, Arlene. (1983). Relating Medicine To Education--A Curriculum Outline. In *Hospice U.S.A.* edited by Austin H. Kutscher, *et al.* New York: Columbia University Press.

Shubin, S. (1978). The Professional Hazard You Face in Nursing. *Nursing* 8(7):25.

SoRelle, Ruth. (1985). Nursing Care for the AIDS Patient Requires Multiple Skills, Strict Adherence to Procedure. *Oncology Times* 7(2): 1-19.

Starr, Paul. (1982). *The Social Transformation of American Medicine.* New York: Basic Books.

Stewart, Sally Ann. (1984). Hospice Care Turns Attention to Children. *USA Today* (October 31): section 6, 5-6.

Torrens, Paul R. (1985). *Hospice Programs and Public Policy.* Chicago, IL: American Hospital Publishing, Inc.

Vachon, M. L. S. (1982). Are Your Patients Burning Out? *Canadian Family Physician* 28:1570-1574.

_____. (1983). Staff Stress in Care of the Terminally Ill in *Hospice Care Principles and Practice,* edited by Charles A. Carr and Donna M. Carr. New York: Springer.

Vachon, M. L. S., W. A. Lyall, and S. J. J. Freeman. (1978). Measurement and Management of Stress in Health Professionals Working with Advanced Cancer Patients. *Death Education* 1:365-375.

Van Fleteren, Frederick. (1983). *Explaining Death To Children.* Brochure. Quakertown, PA: Ever-Kare, Inc.

Wald, Florence S., Zelda Foster, and Henry J. Wald. (1980). The Hospice Movement As A Health Care Reform. *Nursing Outlook* 28(3):173-178.

Ward, B. J. (1978). Hospice Home Care Program. *Nursing Outlook* 26(10):646-49.

Worby, Cyril M., Karen S. Blackman, and John Schneider. (1978). Hospice Care: Current Status and Future Prospects. *Patient Counseling and Health Education* 6(4):61-63.

Zimmerman, Jack M. (1981). *Hospice: Complete Care For The Terminally Ill.* Baltimore-Munich: Urban and Schwarzenberg.

A PERSONAL NOTE

As a public health nurse, my dream through the years was to be able to spend more time with the patient and family in order to provide an individualized and specialized type of care. With ten patients to see within a six-and-a-half hour period, I could only perform the specific treatment of care and travel on to the next home. I spent very little time with the family and as soon as the medication regime was completed or the wound healed, the patient was discharged. According to the dictates of strict professionalism, I could not become deeply involved; I could never really know or address the underlying problems or deeper needs for fear of becoming too emotionally involved with patients.

In nursing school we were trained to *cure* illness; when a patient became very ill with an incurable disease no one wanted to face the situation. We felt guilty for being unable to change an impossible circumstance. Consequently that patient was often left alone; few nurses visited and no one felt comfortable with the terminal patient and his or her family.

Six years ago, my family and I helplessly watched my father die. After the sudden death of my husband as well, I knew I must make a commitment to helping others in similar circumstances.

We valued the time we spent with my dad and we tried to make his life as fruitful as possible, facing each day as a miracle. We knew that fully living in the present would ensure that his past would be held in good stead and that the future would take care of itself.

In contrast, the unfinished business which enveloped me after my husband's death led to a feeling that I never wanted to see an accountant or a lawyer again. I knew then how helpful a group such as hospice could be in assisting families to prepare for an inevitable death. As stated by Carolyn Fitzpatrick, a hospice executive: "Hospice work is joyous because we are given the privilege of knowing that a life is coming to an end. And that gives us all sorts of freedom to help the person who is dying live as he or she wants to live in the time that remains. When someone has an accident or there is an unexpected death, no one has the chance to change anything, or do anything differently in his life" (*Hospice Letter*, 1984).

Because the health care system has traditionally been concerned with curing those who are ill, the emotional and physical needs of those who have no hope of recovery have generally been neglected. This situation has changed somewhat with the widespread adoption of hospice which provides care and emotional support to the dying and their families during the final days of life. Nurses are in a unique position for assessing these needs over a period of time and for planning the patient's care based on their assessments. Nurses have the responsibility to act as catalysts of communication between the physician, patient, family, and significant others.

As an advocate of home health care and with my experiences as a visiting nurse, I quickly learned that "Home is where the heart is" whether home is a house, apartment, residence club, mansion, or shanty when one is ill or well. Sadly enough, there is a widespread feeling that home is for healthy people, while institutions are for sick people. In the past, people have been removed from their homes where they felt most comfortable to be treated in unfamiliar and often frightening surroundings. Only recently has this trend begun to be reversed and the literal "homecoming" of health-related in-home services has been both praised and criticized. More people are dying at home. Hospice allows this to happen with the supportive team. The dying have a right to a great many things that hospitals and nursing homes simply cannot provide. They need life around them, spiritual and emotional comfort, and support of every sort. They need so-called "unsanitary" things, like a favorite dog lying at the foot of the bed. They need their own clothes, their own pictures, music, food, people they know and love, and people they can trust to care about them. Hospices can provide this in their inpatient units but for many individuals and their families it is much better to be at home.

Hospice symbolizes a yearning for a change in value systems to honor the individual and to demonstrate a personal caring. Its roots go far back, its services grounded in the establishment of a caring community and the humanizing of the health care system draws upon common sense, common courtesy, and modern knowledge. Hospice care for the dying is clearly a concept that is in touch with the pulse of our times.

The growth of interest in hospice may be attributed to the social reevaluation of the past few decades that removed from our culture many long-standing taboos, leaving attention to individual dignity and individual rights. Death is now viewed as a natural biological event. Hospice offers a visible alternative to the inflexibility and impersonality of traditional medical-surgical treatment of patients/families, especially the terminally ill. Most important to the hospice concept is emotional accessibility, or the art of being fully present to another human being. As an adherent of the hospice philosophy, I will continue to argue for hospice care as an essential approach to the terminally ill.

Human beings have one great asset over all other living things, and that is that they have free choice. In the course of a terminal illness, a patient can give up, demand attention, and become a total invalid long before it is necessary. A patient can displace anger and a sense of unfairness onto others and make their lives miserable. Or a patient has the choice to complete his or her work, to function in whatever way he or she is capable, and thereby touch many lives by a valiant struggle and a personal sense of purpose. Those patients and families who have allowed me to become a part of their lives through mutual sharing and caring have provided me with additional knowledge as well as a sense of personal satisfaction in hospice work.

Our hospice program was started because of an identified need in the community. A group of committed, loyal, and ambitious citizens who saw this need--many of whom had loved ones who died of terminal illness--set out to accomplish a mission. At that time I was contacted as an administrator of a home health agency to become a part of the movement which has been most rewarding and continues to inspire many aspects of my career both clinically and academically.

Mr. B., my first hospice patient, was in a nursing home dying of lung cancer. The social worker and I spent many long hours with him together and as individuals. We took him for rides, and invited him to join us for a couple of beers regularly along with his friends. One day I remember that he and his two lady friends joined me at the pool; they watched me swim and enjoyed every minute. When Mr. B. had to be hospitalized he became very anxious for he knew everything was not right with his family. The social worker and I knew he and his son had a "falling out" years ago and we understood his need for a reconciliation since his remaining days were limited. After several days of planning and discussions, a phone call was made. I heard: "Son, how are you? I'm not well and need to see you. Let us forget the past, I love you. Can you come?"

The following week the son arrived and sufficient words were exchanged to lead to mutual forgiveness. Mr. B. died five days later. What a first experience! Since then, I've shared both grief and pleasure with innumerable families in similar situations. Each family has a special memory when the imminence of death was translated into painful but loving conversations. In many cases, hospice opened the door for such communication.

With the guidance of the hospice team, patients can face terminal illness with courage, peace, and equanimity. Our role in their struggle is simply that of a catalyst; we can share a moment, a tear perhaps, a hope, a listening ear, and most of all the palliative care to comfort them. Home care is always possible when there is a support system available. It requires very little time on our part to be the facilitator and the catalyst of such a constructive, positive choice. No matter what basic model for hospice is used, home care is an essential component in combination with an inpatient hospice unit.

My experiences with hospice have helped me grow both personally and professionally. I have learned much about people and the impact of illness on family, friends, and the community. I have found satisfaction in working with hospice patients and at the same time gained insights into the various components of hospice organization, administration, staffing, services, and finances. From the involvement with patients and their families, I became more aware of the individual staff requirements for hospice care, that is, flexibility in terms of time schedules, as well as in approach to patient care, the deep commitment to the concept and program, the need for a warm, compassionate personality, reliability in terms of quality of care, and self-awareness in terms of grief, bereavement, and the death and dying concept. The knowledge gained from my "hands-on" experience--as well as in my role as an RN administrator of hospice--could not have been learned in the classroom. Training alone without experience is not sufficient for becoming a good hospice worker or administrator. I am now also better able to educate my students, based on my own training and personal experiences. Hospice administrators must be trained to manage change and must never settle for mediocrity in service provision.

APPENDICES

Appendix A

ACCEPTANCE OF PATIENT/FAMILY CARE POLICIES (ADMISSION CRITERIA)

Patients and their families are accepted for hospice care on the basis of the following:

- Patient has a diagnosis of terminal illness (with a prognosis of six months or less to live).

- Willingness to participate in a physician-directed interdisciplinary program of care.

- A reasonable expectation that the patient's medical, nursing, social, and spiritual needs can be met adequately by the hospice team either by direct services from hospice or referral to existing services in the community.

- The patient's qualified physician is involved in the program of care.

- Hospice care follows a written plan of treatment established by the interdisciplinary team with continued supervision by the physician who certifies and recertifies the care and treatment plan as needed but at least every thirty days.

- Cooperative attitude of patient and/or family with ability to participate in patient and family care.

Patients are accepted without regard to color, race, religious creed, lifestyle, handicap, ancestry, national origin, union membership, age, or sex.

Appendix B

Development of Plan of Care

A written plan of care is established initially upon admission and is maintained through the ongoing assessment mechanism to ensure implementation. The care plan is established by the attending physician, medical director, and interdisciplinary team prior to admission for care and is certified in writing with attending physician signature at least every thirty days thereafter as long as services are provided and at any time when additions or changes occur. The plan of care must include:

- Assessment of the patient's and family's needs including medical, nursing, functional, and psychosocial status and identification of the services, including the management of discomfort and symptom relief

- Diagnosis and prognosis

- Scope, type, and frequency of services, treatment, and medications needed to meet the patient's and family's needs based on identification of problems and goals from the assessment

- Identification of person/persons responsible for each service

- Follow-up to determine if goals were met, or partially met and reassessment as needed.

The plan is reviewed and updated as necessary but at least every two weeks by the interdisciplinary team (IDG). The IDG team, however, meets weekly to review and update the plan of care on each patient. This review and update is documented through minutes of IDG meetings with signatures of those attending including the signature of the medical director.

In summary, the plan of care developed in consultation with the hospice staff and IDG team covers all pertinent diagnoses, including mental status, types of services, and equipment required, frequency of visits, prognosis, rehabilitation potential, functional limitations, activities permitted, nutritional requirements, medications and treatments, any safety measures to protect against injury, instructions for timely discharge or referral, and any other appropriate items. If a physician refers a patient under a plan of treatment which cannot be completed until after an evaluation visit, the physician is consulted to approve additions or modifications to the original plan. Orders for therapy services include the specific procedures and modalities to be used and the amount, frequency, and duration.

Conformance with Physician's Orders

Drugs and treatments are administered by hospice staff only as ordered by the physician. The nurse or therapist immediately records and signs oral orders and obtains the physician's countersignature. Hospice staff check all medications a patient may be taking to identify possible ineffective drug therapy or adverse reactions, significant side effects, drug allergies, and contraindicated medication, and promptly report any problems to the physician.

Continuity of Care

Hospice assures the continuity of patient/family care in home, outpatient, and inpatient settings. This is accomplished through defining the expected role of the family in providing care when appropriate. Also, the hospice care team retains the responsibility for determining the appropriate location for treatment. However, the hospice care team must consult with the family about changes in the treatment setting and provide necessary information to facilitate the transfer of the patient from an inpatient to a home setting or the reverse.

Ongoing assessment of patient/family needs is carried out by the hospice care team through prompt development and review of the interdisciplinary group plan of care and provision of adequate and appropriate patient/family information at the point of transfer between care settings.

Continuation of Patient/Family Care Policies

Each patient/family is admitted by a nurse for home nursing assessment following medical evaluation. A medical social worker is then assigned for ongoing psychosocial evaluation. Based on the initial medical, nursing, and social worker assessment other team members are assigned. The *RN serves as the coordinator of services*. The staff members initially assigned continue to serve the patient/family. If coverage is needed, the primary staff nurse is responsible for any additional assignments or changes in assignment through the nursing supervisor.

- Patient care is continued on basis of need and in accordance with physician recertification.

- Specific medical/nursing orders are verified by the physician responsible for the medical care of the patient; for example, order and dosage for chemotherapeutic drugs must be obtained prior to each dosage based on results of bloodwork which is done the day prior to chemotherapy administration. The hospice RN is responsible for obtaining these orders in writing directly from the physician.

- Nursing orders are carried out according to physician certification and hospice procedure, for example, Hickman catheter, Cormed pump. (See specific written procedures.)

- Skilled astute assessment must be made daily on each patient. Any changes must be reported to the physician immediately. A written summary is submitted to the physician and fiscal intermediary with each certification/recertification.

Hospice assures that the RN doing a treatment knows how or will be appropriately trained to do the procedure through the agency as authoritative source. The same policy and principle pertains to all hospice care team members.

Patient Care Coverage and Coordination Policy

- Upon acceptance of a patient/family assignment, the primary care person (RN, physical therapist, or speech therapist) must report status of patient to nursing coordinators/supervisors daily and on Friday afternoons for weekend/holiday coverage. Additional reports must be given as condition changes, but at least weekly each Friday afternoon.

- Weekly report meetings for primary care persons are held in the hospice office. If any staff primary care person cannot be present, a telephone call must be made to discuss status of all patients/families. Medical social workers must also attend or provide a report by telephone. All other hospice care team members are encouraged to attend this patient care conference.

- In addition, each hospice care team member must report to the primary care person on a regular basis but at least once weekly on Friday.

- Daily itineraries *must* be in the central office for all staff assignments. Daily schedules can be called in for those team members who are not scheduled to be in the office.

- The assigned hospice care team will meet to discuss admission of patient no later than seven to ten days after admission of the patient. In addition, all admissions are discussed at the weekly IDG meeting.

Appendix C

The purpose of the patient grievance procedure is to resolve allegations of discrimination. This procedure incorporates standards of due process and provides for an equitable resolution of complaints. Due process includes the following:

- A process and time frame for filing a grievance
- An initial hearing
- A process and time frame for appeal
- Options for resolution
- Process for the maintenance and availability of records
- Process for confidentiality
- Auxiliary aids, including interpreters, for communication with the employee or beneficiary.

The following steps should be taken if a patient/family wishes to voice grievance. The goal is to accommodate the wishes and maintain the dignity and happiness of each individual regardless of age, sex, race, color, creed, national origin, handicap, marital status, or political affiliation.

Step 1. If a patient/family expresses a grievance to an employee, the employee will *immediately* transmit this to his or her immediate supervisor who will then immediately report this information to the administrator as coordinator.

Step 2. The administrator will then meet with the patient/family within a twenty-four hour period of time encouraging the individual to voice his or her problems and assuring the patient of his or her rights.

Step 3. Corrective measures will be made immediately, whenever possible on all valid complaints.

Step 4. If the administrator feels it would be beneficial to the patient/family, another professional or family member will be invited to discuss the problem and help resolve it.

Step 5. If corrective action, for whatever reason, cannot be taken immediately by the administrator, a written complaint must be filed with the administrator and chairman of the board of directors.

Step 6. A hearing must be held within seven days before the executive committee.

Step 7. A decision is then made by the executive committee.

Step 8. If the decision is not agreeable to the patient/family, an appeal must be filed immediately after the hearing.

Step 9. The executive committee and administrator must then provide options for resolution within seven days. (The entire process must not exceed fourteen days.)

Step 10. A decision must be agreed upon within a *total* of fourteen days from time of initial complaint to complete resolution.

Records regarding complaints are maintained by the administrator who provides availability of records upon written request to insure confidentiality. The agency's attorney is consulted for legal aspects as needed. Appropriate auxiliary aids to persons with impaired sensory, manual, or speaking skills are provided to afford such persons an equal opportunity for communication. A description of some of the auxiliary aids follows.

- Arrangement to share a TTY (teletypewriter) line

- Services of qualified sign language interpreters

- Braille copies of hospice brochure, nondiscrimination policy, and consent form

- Tape recordings of the hospice brochure, nondiscrimination policy, and consent form

- Flash cards in large print of hospice information

- Pictogram and scriptogram pamphlets

- Braille copies of hospice information available at Association for the Blind and Office for Physically Disabled

- Braille machine from hospice's pharmacy consultant available for hospice staff, patient, and family use
- Coordinated interpreter service
- State School for Deaf services

Appendix D

HOSPICE OF NORTHEASTERN PENNSYLVANIA PROTOCOL: CONTINUOUS
SUBCUTANEOUS MORPHINE INFUSION UTILIZING CORMED PUMP

Developed by Dawn Hannon, R.N. and Sharon Wrobel, R.N., Hospice of PA, Inc., March 1984.

The Cormed Pump, a battery-operated device slightly larger than a transistor radio, delivers medication at a continuous, predetermined rate. Capable of delivering 20cc to 53.5cc of medication in a 24-hour period, it has been used for at-home administration of morphine, both intravenously via a Hickman catheter, and subcutaneously via #23 butterfly. It is also utilized for administering chemotherapy directly into the hepatic artery.

Equipment Needed:

- Cormed infusion pump with power pack
- Rate meter and screwdriver
- 50cc. disposable Reservoir Bag and tubing
- SC. morphine sulfate solution--(15mg./cc. or prescribed strength)
- IM Narcan solution (0.1 mg./cc.)
- Sterile 50cc. syringe with needle
- Sterile 3cc. syringes (2) with needles
- Alcohol swabs, Betadine swabs
- #23 butterfly
- Hypoallergenic tape

Preparation

1. Instruct patient and family re: use of Cormed equipment; use and precautions related to morphine; and Narcan emergency use.

2. Cleanse top of vial(s) containing morphine solution with alcohol swab.

3. Remove needle protector from 50cc. syringe.

4. Using sterile technique, insert needle into vial and withdraw desired amount of morphine solution into the 50cc. syringe; replace needle protector.

5. Remove needle protector from 3cc. syringe.

6. Using sterile technique, draw up .5cc. morphine solution into the 3cc. syringe; replace needle protector.

7. Fill 50cc. Reservoir Bag (morphine solution and Bag should be at room temperature to facilitate expelling of air).

A) Using aseptic technique, disconnect long tubing from Reservoir Bag at proximal connection site--keep ends of Reservoir Bag tubing sterile.

B) Remove needle from prefilled (morphine) 50cc. syringe.

C) Connect syringe to Reservoir Bag at the proximal connection and fill the bag with the morphine solution.

D) Expel all air from Reservoir Bag and short tubing.

E) Reattach long tubing to Reservoir Bag at the proximal connection.

F) Remove distal end cap from tubing and expel all remaining air; replace distal end cap; clamp tubing near distal end.

8. Have Narcan solution and 3cc. syringe readily available for (IM) administration in the event that adverse reaction to morphine occurs.

9. Remove protective cap from luerlok end of butterfly, attach 3cc. syringe with 0.5cc. MS, flush air from butterfly tubing. Leave syringe attached.

10. Adjust pump to correct flow rate using rate meter as per manufacturer's instructions.

Procedure

(STERILE TECHNIQUE MUST BE MAINTAINED THROUGHOUT)

1. Choose site for needle insertion on abdomen.

2. Swab area with Betadine, then with alcohol.

3. Remove needle protector from #23 butterfly, insert subcutaneously into abdomen, checking to be sure needle isn't in vein.

4. Coil tubing and tape to abdomen securely.

5. Remove syringe from end of butterfly, connect distal end of Cormed tubing, unclamp tubing. (Tape connection as safety precaution).

6. Turn pump on (noise pump makes is minimal).

7. Check flow rate with rate meter for accuracy.
*OBSERVE PATIENT FOR ANY ADVERSE REACTION.

8. Secure pump in harness to patient or to bed.

9. Insertion site may be dressed with occlusive transparent dressing if desired.

Notes

1. Change butterfly needle and site every 3 days. Observe for signs of local irritation or infection.

2. Reservoir bag and tubing must be changed at least weekly.

3. Power pack must be changed weekly (recharge for minimum of 16 hours.)

4. Formula for calculating flow rate percent:

x mgm MS/hr - mgm MS/cc

7 mgm MS/hr - 7.5 mgm MS/cc = 0.93 cc/hr

0.93 cc/hr x 24 hrs. = 22.3 cc/24 hrs.

22.3 cc - 53.5 (capacity of pump) = 41.8%

HICKMAN CATHETER PROCEDURES: PATIENT TEACHING GUIDELINES

Irrigating the Hickman Catheter

Irrigation is done daily through the adaptor (injectable) cap. Aseptic technique throughout.

1. Wash hands.

2. Assemble equipment on a clean, dry surface:

    a. 1 - 10cc syringe

    b. 1 - #20 needle

    c. 1 - #25 needle

    d. Heparin/saline solution 100 U/cc

    e. Alcohol swab

3. Draw up 10cc heparinized saline 100 U/cc into syringe using #20 needle.

4. Aspirate air, change to #25 needle.

5. Clean adaptor cap with alcohol swab - allow to air dry.

6. Insert #25 needle into center of cap; *slowly* infuse 8cc of the heparin.

7. Withdraw needle; discard syringe with remaining 2cc heparin.

RATIONALE:

> Rapid flushing and/or complete emptying of syringe may create a vacuum, causing a back flow of blood into the catheter tip, which may cause clotting in the catheter.

8. Curl, don't kink, catheter and tape securely to chest.

Hickman Care Insertion Site Protocol

This protocol is substituted for sterile dressing changes two weeks after Hickman catheter is inserted.

1. Wash hands.

2. Assemble supplies on a clean, dry surface:

    occlusive transparent dressing or similar dsg.

    alcohol, Betadine swabs

    tape

3. Remove and discard old dressing. Inspect site for redness, irritation or discharge.

4. With Betadine swab, cleanse area around insertion site in ever widening circles.

5. Repeat step #4 with alcohol swab, allow to air dry.

6. Cover site with occlusive transparent dressing or other dsg.

7. Curl, don't kink, catheter and tape securely to chest wall.

Drawing Blood from the Hickman Catheter

Equipment:

1. Appropriate clamp

2. Sterile 5cc syringe

3. Sterile 10cc syringe filled with 10cc heparin-saline solution (100U/cc)

4. Sterile syringe with needle--appropriate size for amount of blood needed

5. Alcohol swab

6. Sterile adaptor cap

7. Sterile lab tube(s)

Procedure:

1. Expose tubing of Hickman catheter.

2. Clamp catheter tubing with clamp about 3" from the connection site.

3. After wiping the connection site with an alcohol swab, disconnect the adaptor cap from the Hickman and discard.

4. With tubing still clamped, attach sterile 5cc syringe to the connection.

5. Unclamp clamp, and withdraw 5cc of blood from the catheter into the syringe.

6. Clamp catheter tubing. Disconnect blood-filled syringe and discard.

7. With Hickman still clamped, attach sterile (empty) syringe to the tubing.

8. Remove clamp from the catheter and withdraw the required amount of blood necessary for lab tests. Clamp catheter tubing.

9. Disconnect blood-filled syringe and set aside.

10. Attach the heparin-filled syringe to the Hickman. Remove clamp and instill 8cc of the solution into the catheter. Clamp catheter.

11. Disconnect 10cc syringe from the catheter and discard.

12. With catheter tubing still clamped, attach sterile adaptor cap to the connection site. Remove clamp.

13. Attach sterile needle to the blood-filled syringe. Insert needle into the rubber top of the lab tube(s), and allow the vacuum to draw the desired amount of blood into the tube.

14. Label lab tube(s): Patient's name, doctor's name, and tests to be done.

15. Tape Hickman catheter securely to patient's skin.

Changing the Injectable Catheter cap

NOTE: If cap is removed for any reason, i.e., drawing blood, it is not to be reused; it is replaced each time it is detached from the catheter. The cap is changed q 2 weeks when the only procedure done is daily irrigation with heparin.

1. Wash hands.

2. Assemble equipment on a clean, dry surface:

   a. Betadine swabs

   b. Alcohol swabs

   c. Adaptor (injectable) cap

   d. Hickman clamp

3. Swab cap/catheter connection, first with Betadine, then with alcohol swabs; place end on alcohol swab or sterile 4 x 4.

4. Clamp catheter 2 - 3 inches away from end.

5. Open package containing new cap, maintaining sterility.

6. Remove old cap.

7. Replace with sterile cap.

8. Tape connection.

9. Unclamp catheter.

10. Curl, don't kink, catheter and tape securely to chest.

Hickman Protocols--(Abbreviated)

Dressing change: done three times weekly. This procedure is substituted for sterile dressing change after two (2) week healing period, post catheter insertion.

1. Wash hands. Carefully remove old dressing.

2. Wash hands.

3. Cleanse area around catheter with alcohol or Betadine swabs in ever widening circles. Observe for placement, redness, irritation.

4. Curl, don't kink, catheter and secure to chest wall with tape or occlusive transparent dsg.

Irrigation: Done daily through injectable catheter cap.

1. Wash hands.

2. Assemble equipment.

3. Draw up 10cc heparinized saline 100U/cc using #20 needle.

4. Aspirate air; change to #25 needle.

5. Clean adaptor cap with alcohol swab--allow to air dry.

6. Slowly infuse 8cc heparin-saline solution.

7. Discard syringe with 2cc solution remaining in it.

RATIONALE:

rapid flushing and/or complete emptying of syringe may create a vacuum, causing a back flow of blood into the catheter tip, which may cause clotting in the catheter.

8. Change cap every two weeks.

Drawing blood:

Note: Clamp between steps, maintain strict aseptic technique.

1. Wash hands.

2. Equipment needed:

2-5cc syringes

1-10cc syringe with 10cc heparin-saline (100U/cc)

lab tubes

injectable catheter

3. Remove and discard injection cap.

4. Clean end of catheter with alcohol swab.

5. With 5cc syringe--withdraw 5cc blood and heparin and discard.

6. With 5cc syringe--or one large enough for specimen needed--withdraw required amount of blood.

7. Slowly irrigate catheter with 8cc heparin.

8. With clamp in place, syringe left in place to insure asepsis, inject blood into appropriate lab tubes; remove syringe and discard remaining 2cc heparin.

9. Clean end of catheter with alcohol.

10. Attach new adaptor cap, remove clamp, tape to catheter securely.

11. Curl catheter and tape to chest wall.

Note: family teaching re daily irrigation and 3 x weekly dressing change, started while in hospital, must be constantly reinforced at home.

Changing injectable catheter cap: (q 2 weeks if no blood drawn)

1. Wash hands.

2. Swab connection with alcohol swab.

3. Clamp catheter.

4. Remove old cap.

5. Replace with sterile cap.

6. Unclamp catheter.

7. Tape securely.

Appendix E

BEREAVEMENT PROGRAM RESOURCES

Developed By Nancy Menapace, Director of Staff Relations and Bereavement Services, Hospice of Pa., Inc., 916 Wyoming Avenue, Scranton, PA 18510

Aries, Philippe. *Western Attitudes Toward Death, From the Middle Ages to the Present.* Baltimore & London: Johns Hopkins University Press, 1974.

Barrett, Carol J. Intimacy in Widowhood. *Psychology of Women Quarterly* 3(1981):473-485.

Barrett, Carol J., and Karen M. Schneweis. An Empirical Search for Stages of Widowhood. *Omega* 2(1980):97-103.

Baum, Martha, and Rainer C. Baum. *Growing Old: A Societal Perspective.* Englewood Cliffs, NJ: Prentice-Hall, 1980.

Bloomfield, Harold H., Melba Colgrove, and Peter McWilliams. *How To Survive the Loss of a Love.* New York: Bantam Books, 1976. 131 p.

Carey, Raymond G. Weathering Widowhood: Problems and Adjustments of the Widowed During the First Year. *Omega* 2(1979):163-173.

Davidson, Glen W. *Living With Dying.* Minneapolis: Augsburg Publishing House, 1975.

Easson, William M. The Family of the Dying Child. *Pediatric Clinics of North America* 19(1972):1157-1165.

Engle, George L. A Group Dynamic Approach to Teaching and Learning about Grief. *Omega* 2(1980):45-59.

258 QUALITY HOSPICE CARE

George, Linda K. *Role Transitions in Later Life*. Monterey, CA: Brooks/Cloe Publishing Company, 1980.

Gergen, Kenneth J., Mary Gergen, Margaret S. Stroebe, and Wolfgang Stroebe. The Broken Heart: Reality or Myth? *Omega* 2(1981-82):87-102.

Grof, Stanisslav, and Joan Halifax. *The Human Encounter with Death*. New York: Dutton, 1977.

Jackson, Edgar N. *Understanding Grief*. Nashville: Abington Press, 1975.

Kastenbaum, Robert J. *Death, Society, & Human Experience*. St. Louis: C. V. Mosby Company, 1977.

Kennell, John H., Marshall H. Klaus, and Howard Slyter. The Mourning Response of Parents to the Death of a Newborn Infant. *The New England Journal of Medicine*, August 1970, pp. 344-349.

Kohn, Jane Burgess, and Willard K. Kohn. *The Widower*. Boston: The Beacon Press, 1978.

Kutscher, Austin H., and Lillian G. Kutscher, eds. *Religion and Bereavement*. New York: Health Sciences Publishing Corporation, 1972.

Lattanzi, Marcie, and Diane Coffelt. *Bereavement Care Manual*. Boulder, CO: Boulder County Hospice, Inc. (2825 Marine Street, Boulder, CO 80303), 1979.

Lindemann, Erich. Symptomatology and Management of Acute Grief. *American Journal of Psychiatry* 101 (September 1944):141-148.

Miller, Jack Silvey. *The Healing Power of Grief*. New York: The Seabury Press, 1979.

Patterson, Robert D. Grief and Depression in Old People. *Maryland State Medical Journal* 18(September 1969):75-79.

Piscus, Lily. *Death and the Family: The Importance of Mourning*. New York: Pantheon Books, 1974.

Riverside, Hospice. *Bereavement: A Guide for Training*. Consumer Health Education, Dept. of Environmental and Community Medicine, College of Medicine and Dentistry of NJ, Rutgers Medical School, Piscataway, NJ, 1981.

Romaniuk, Michael, and J. Michael Priddy. Widowhood Peer Counseling. *Counseling and Values* April 1980, pp. 195-202.

Saunders, Catherine M. Comparison of Younger and Older Spouses in Bereavement Outcome. *Omega* 11(1980-81):217-231.

Shepard, Martin. *Someone You Love is Dying: A Guide for Helping and Coping.* New York: Harmony Books, 1975. 219 p.

Shwartz, L. H., and J. L. Schwartz. *The Psychodynamics of Patient Care.* Englewood Cliffs, NJ: Prentice-Hall, 1972.

Tanner, Ira J. *The Gift of Grief.* New York: Hawthorn Books, 1976. 167 p.

U.S. Department of Health and Human Services, Public Health Services. *Talking to Children About Death.* Public Inquiries, National Institute of Mental Health (5600 Fishers Lane, Rockville, MD 20857) 1979.

Wass, Hannelore. *Dying: Facing the Facts.* Washington, New York, & London: Hemisphere Publishing, 1979.

Weisman, Avery D. Is mourning necessary? In A.C. Carr, H. Goldberg, A.H. Kutcher, D. Peretz, and B. Schoerberg (Eds.) *Anticipatory Grief.* New York: Columbia University Press, 1974.

York, Janet B., and Sanford A. Weinstein. The Effect of a Videotape about Death on Bereaved Children in Family Therapy. *Omega* 4(1980-81):355-361.

Appendix F

Introduction

The hospice philosophy has always acknowledged the significant impact of grief and the need to continue to offer services to the bereaved families. Grief is a normal response to loss; however, it is the strongest emotion experienced in a lifetime and receives little or no social support. Grief has been deritualized and many times the survivors are left without direction or norms to guide them through this crisis period in their lives. The bereavement program at Hospice of Pa., Inc. addresses the needs of the bereaved families by one-to-one visitation, phone calls, written correspondence, workshops, and memorial services. The program provides information, education, support, and counseling to the families, and provides continued information about the bereaved families to the direct care team. The goal is to act as a bridge back to the community. The bereavement program is implemented by the continuing care team which is supervised by a professional bereavement counselor and staffed by trained volunteers.

Referrals

1. All families of deceased hospice patients are referred to the continuing care team for follow-up.

2. Families who have been evaluated as high-risk survivors prior to the death of the hospice patient are referred to the continuing care team for intervention by the bereavement counselor.

Referrals: After the Death of the Patient

1. Referrals are made by the direct care team to the bereavement counselor at the weekly interdisciplinary group meeting.

2. All members of the direct care team help in evaluating the bereaved family.

3. Low-risk survivors are assigned to a volunteer member of the continuing care team.

4. High-risk survivors are assigned to the bereavement counselor.

Referrals: High-Risk Survivors

1. The goal is to have the majority of the high-risk survivors evaluated and referred prior to the death of the hospice patient. This provides additional support to the patient/family and direct care staff during the crisis of dying and death, and gives the opportunity to provide the necessary trust relationship between the family and the bereavement counselor.

2. High-risk survivors are:

• those who have a psychiatric history and/or multiple crises at the time of the death

• those caring for an ill or dying person for over six months

• those with no previous grief experience

• those without available support from family, friends, or faith belief

• those evaluated by the instrument developed by C.M. Parkes. (See instrument which follows.) High-risk survivors are those evaluated with a score of over 14.

• those who are experiencing the negative effect of anticipatory grief: completion of grieving with emotional and/or physical detachment and abandonment from the patient.

A guideline to "the rule of thirds." Approximately one third of all survivors need professional counseling, one third need extra support, and one third will survive with or without extra support.

BEREAVEMENT ASSESSMENT - REFERRAL
(C. M. Parkes)

Name of Bereaved_____Age_____

Address_____ Home Phone_____

Relationship to Deceased _____ Date of Death_____

Short Description of Circumstances of Death

_____

_____

_____

Primary Caregiver interested in follow-up?   _____Yes   _____No

Staff Members Closely Involved:

Nurse_____ Phone_____

Volunteer_____ Phone_____

Other (please specify)_____ Phone_____

Intended Role in Follow-Up_____ Phone_____

Others needing follow-up (indicate name, relationship, phone):   _____None

_____

_____

_____

Questions: (circle one item in each section)

A. Age of Primary Caregiver

1. 75+
2. 66 - 75
3. 56 - 65
4. 46 - 55
5. 15 - 45

B. Occupation of principal wage earner in a primary caregivers' family

1. Professional & Executive
2. Semi-Professional
3. Office & Clerical
4. Semi-skilled Manual
5. Unskilled Manual

C. Length of primary caregiver's preparation for patient's death

1. Fully prepared for long time
2. Fully prepared for less than 2 weeks
3. Partially prepared
4. Totally unprepared

D. Clinging or Pining

1. Never   4. Frequent
2. Seldom   5. Constant
3. Moderate   6. Constant and Intense

E. Anger

1. None (normal) 2. Mild irritation   3. Moderate, occasional outbursts
4. Severe, spoiling relationships   5. Extreme, always bitter

		Questionnaire
F. Self Reproach		Summary

F. Self Reproach
  1. None   4. Severe, preoccupational,
  2. Mild, vague & general   self blame   A.
  3. Moderate, some   5. Extreme, major
                                  problem   B.

G. Family   C.
  1. Warm, will give   4. Not supportive
       full support   5. No family   D.
  2. Doubtful
  3. Supportive but live at distance   E.

H. How will Primary Caregiver Cope?   F.
  1. Well   Normal grief and recovery without special
                help.   G.
  2. Fair   Probably manage without special help.
  3. Doubtful   May need special help.   H.
  4. Badly   Requires special help.
  5. Very badly Requires urgent help.   Total =

Potentially Destructive Behaviors Observed

_____
_____
_____

Details of Help Already Being Given (include information regarding available support systems)

_____
_____
_____

Comments

_____
_____
_____

_____
Signature

_____

_____
Date

Overall Procedure for Visitation

The visitation procedure can be addressed both informally by the direct care team, and formally by the continuing care team. The informal visitation by the direct care team includes the visit with the family at the death and during the funeral proceedings. These visits, and all other follow-up visits, are to meet the needs of the family and the direct care team member.

Formally, the continuing care team will receive referrals from the direct care team and make arrangements for the initial visit. A request can be made by the direct care team member at any time during the care of the patient to have a member of the continuing care team visit the family. The direct care team member may request this visit for several reasons:

1. The family requests to talk with someone about the death and the bereavement period.

2. The family appears to be having great difficulty with facing the prospects of grief, and counseling at this time may be beneficial.

3. The direct care team member believes it would be helpful for the continuing care team member to meet the patient and the family prior to the bereavement period. The continuing care team member can be introduced as a member of the hospice staff; it is not necessary to introduce the team member as part of the continuing care team.

A feasible procedure for referral from the direct care team to the continuing care team is a biweekly continuing care team meeting. At this meeting the direct care team member presents a verbal and written referral of all his or her patients that have died since the last meeting.

It is hoped that verbalizing the experience that the direct care member had with the dying patient and the family will also be beneficial. This will provide the direct care team member an opportunity to receive support and positive feedback from the continuing care team. Also, open communication of this nature will enhance the hospice team as a whole.

The rationale for someone other than the direct care team member being involved in the bereavement period is:

1. The hospice concept emphasizes the importance of grief and that this is a difficult period of adjustment.

2. The hospice direct care team member is also experiencing a degree of loss when the death occurs; this can make the bereavement intervention very difficult. Also the direct care team members become involved with new referrals to the hospice program and time and energy are placed elsewhere.

3. Obsessional review or "telling their story," as reported by R. Kastenbaum in his book, *Death, Society, and Human*

Experience, is recognized as a necessary part of the grief process.* It appears to be easier for the bereaved family member to relate the telling of the story to someone who has not been involved with the care of the dying patient.

Procedure for Initiating Visitation

After the referral has been made an initial assessment is made as to whether the bereaved is a "high risk" survivor or will experience a normal grief process. The initial assessment is made from the report given by the direct care team. One instrument for this assessment is the Bereavement Assessment-Referral (see pages 263-264) and, of course, the verbal report given by the direct care team member. "High risk" survivors are:

1. Those caring for an ill or dying person longer than six months.

2. Those with no previous experience with bereavement.

3. Those without available support from family, friends, and faith.

4. Those who appear depressed, stricken, and angry one to two months after the death--no struggle to survive.

5. Those who displayed an unstable emotional state prior to the death of the loved one.

At this point the bereaved family that has been assessed as "normal" survivors are assigned to a volunteer. Those assessed as "high risk" survivors will be visited by the bereavement counselor.

The continuing care team makes arrangements for the initial visit. A bereavement package that includes helpful information is prepared. Suggestions for this package are:

1. A form with the volunteer's name and telephone number and visitation procedure.

2. A pamphlet explaining that grief is a normal process and normal experience in the time of bereavement.

3. A listing and description of community services and available references; this should also include basic information about home care assistance and repairs and maintenance.

4. Information about the educational workshop.

---

* Kastenbaum, Robert. *Death, Society and Human Experience.* St. Louis, MO: C.V. Mosby, 1977.

The continuing care team will further assess the grief process of the bereaved family member. If referral is necessary this can be done at this time. Those bereaved persons that are open to visitation will then receive a visit three months, six months, and twelve months after the death of their loved one. The initial visit is made within the first two weeks after the death and when the referral is received. Thus a total of four visits will be made to the home. For those persons that are assessed as "high risk" survivors visits will be made as necessary.

Telephone calls and written notes are part of the visitation program. A telephone call is made one week after the first visit, on holidays, anniversaries, and birthdays. The bereaved person is asked to call the continuing care team member when they feel it is necessary.

The continuing care team member will use the bereavement initial assessment report and the bereavement progress notes. The bereavement initial assessment report is used on the initial visit. The continuing care team member acquires this information through an informal interview technique, not a question and answer period. Care is taken to enter each visit and communication between the continuing care team member and the bereaved person on the bereavement progress notes. The continuing care team also contacts the direct care team member that referred the bereaved family after each visit and when they think it would be helpful.

Specific Procedure for Visitation by the Continuing Care Team

Purpose

1. To provide support for the bereaved.

2. To give necessary information to the bereaved.

3. To provide the direct care team with continuing information about the bereaved family.

4. To assess if referrals are necessary.

5. To receive and communicate any information that may be helpful to the hospice team in general.

Time

All bereaved families are to be contacted and receive a visit within the first two weeks after the death of the family member. Follow-up visits are suggested at three months, six months, and one year. Phone calls and written communication are indicated on holidays, anniversaries, and as necessary. A follow-up phone call is indicated within a week after the first visit.

Referrals

All referrals will be received via the bereavement counselor. The bereavement counselor receives the referral from the direct care team member. All high risk survivors will be visited by the bereavement counselor. All other referrals may be visited by the continuing care team volunteer.

Initial Contact

The initial contact is made by phone. Introductions are made and arrangements are made for a visitation. The initial introduction can be similar to the following: "Hello, I am with the hospice continuing care team. We like to keep in contact with our families. How are you doing? --- What is the best time for me to stop and see you?"

Visitation

1. A continuing care team pamphlet is given to each bereaved family.

2. A good opening is a sentence using: "What and How in the Here and Now."

3. Be a good listener.

4. Assess needs:

    a. Medical, physical, social, emotional, and spiritual

    b. Housekeeping

    c. Available support from family and friends

    d. Insurance

    e. If the bereaved has experienced grief

    f. What is difficult for the bereaved

    g. What are the main concerns of the bereaved

    h. Job

5. Do not force disclosure of feelings.

6. Self disclosure, for the volunteer, is curvilinear in nature: too little or too much is not helpful to the bereaved.

7. Assess potential for depression and suicide:

    a. Probe further if the bereaved discusses their own death;

    b. If so, assess if the bereaved has thoughts of suicide;

c. Is there a plan?

d. Is it lethal?

If the above conditions are present with the possibility of suicide, contact the bereavement counselor, hospice, a family member, or a family physician before leaving the home. Talking about suicide *cannot* initiate the thought of suicide or be harmful to the bereaved.

8. Ascertain if the bereaved was satisfied with the hospice care and if they desire a visit with the physician who attended the deceased.

Post Visit

1. Record only necessary nonconfidential information in the bereavement notes.

2. Contact the bereavement counselor.

3. Contact the direct care team nurse.

4. Complete bereavement initial assessment report.

Additional Information

As a rule we do not give advice; however,

1. Let them know it is all right to grieve.

2. To make as few changes as possible during the first year of grief.

3. Assure them we are available at all times.

Appendix G

It is agreed that as a member of the Hospice of Pennsylvania, Inc. Continuing Care Team, I will commit for the period of one year's time to assume the following responsibilities:

Complete the initial volunteer training program.

Complete the bereavement team training program.

Regular attendance at the Continuing Care Team meetings.

Visit bereaved families as assigned by the Bereavement Coordinator.

Continuing care will include the following: supportive measures, assessment, and intervention strategies.

Chart all interactions and record them at the Hospice of Pennsylvania, Inc. office.

Use sound judgement and request clinical backup from the Bereavement Coordinator when indicated, or when questions or concerns arise.

Request supervision or information when needed.

In addition, I agree to give Hospice of Pennsylvania thirty days notice of resignation from the program.

Signed:

_____   _____
Continuing Care Team Member   Date

_____   _____
Bereavement Coordinator   Date

Appendix H

Hospice of Pennsylvania, Inc. Continuing Care Team

Hospice understands the pain of bereavement. We are here to help you.

We would like adjustment after the death of a loved one to be like this,

However, the process of adjustment is,

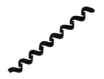

Make as few changes as possible the first year

Grief is a *normal* response to loss. Some normal grief reactions are:

- a need to cry
- a need to sigh

- a need to "tell your story" time and time again
- a feeling of searching and yearning
- an empty feeling
- a sense of presence of your loved one
- difficulty in concentrating
- a feeling of disorganization
- restlessness
- irritability
- loss of appetite
- insomnia
- weight loss

ALLOW YOURSELF TO MOURN

You are invited to attend a workshop about grief and loss. A member of our team will get in touch with you about the date and time. We hope you can join us.

Please call us if you have any questions or if you would just like to talk.

Call _____
or
Hospice office: 961-0725

Bibliography

Amenta, Madalon. (1984). Reimbursement, accreditation and the movement's future: hospice has initiated reform, but will it be lasting. *The American Journal of Hospice Care* 1(1):10-14.

American Hospital Association. (1984). *Outreach* 5(4): entire issue.

_____. (1984). Washington report. Hospice programs move slowly to seek Medicare certification. *Outreach* 5(2):4.

Ames, Richard P. (1980). Starting a hospice requires tenacity, high standards. *Hospital Progress* 61:56-59.

Argyris, Chris. (1957). *Personality and Organization.* New York: Harper and Bros.

_____. (1964). *Integrating the Individual and the Organization.* New York: John Wiley and Sons.

Aries, Philippe. (1974). *Western Attitudes Toward Death.* Baltimore: Johns Hopkins University Press.

Armado, Anthony J. (1980). *Chairman of the NHO Committee on Reimbursement and Licensure, Annual Report to the Membership of the National Hospice Organization.* McLean, VA: National Hospice Organization.

Bellamy, Carol. (1984). Paper presented at the Columbia University Seminar on Health Care: At What Cost?, New York, April 27th.

Berger-Friedman, Patricia J. (1983). Paying for Hospice Care. *Hospitals* 57(16):106-108.

Blum, John D., and Dennis A. Robbins. (1982). Regulation. *Hospitals* 56(23):91-94, 96.

Brooks, Charles H., and Kathleen Smyth-Staruch. (1983). *Cost Savings Of Hospice Home Care To Third-Party Insurers.* Cleveland, OH: Hospice Council for Northern Ohio, Blue Cross of Northeast Ohio, and Case Western Reserve University.

Bunn, Elizabeth G. (1984). Volunteers as the backbone. *The American Journal of Hospice Care* 1(1):34-36.

Califano, Jose G. (1978). Address to the National Hospice Organization's First Annual Banquet, Washington, DC, October 5th.

Carr, Charles A., and Donna M. Carr. (1983). *Hospice Care Principles and Practice.* New York: Springer Publishing Company.

Caudill, William. (1957). *The Psychiatric Hospital As A Small Society.* Cambridge, MA: Harvard University Press.

Centers for Disease Control. (1985). Telephone conference with author, May 6th.

Clark, Matt, Mariana Gasnell, and Deborah Witherspoon. (1982). AIDS: A Lethal Mystery Story. *Newsweek* (Dec. 27): 63-64.

Clifford, Anne. (1979). Children With Cancer Life-Oriented. *Scranton Times* (PA). April 20th.

Cohen, Kenneth P. (1979). *Hospice Prescription for Terminal Care.* Rockville, MD: Aspen Systems Corporation.

Congressional Record. (1978). Intent description regarding terminal illness by Senators Edward M. Kennedy, Robert Dole, and Abraham Ribicoff. May 18th.

Connecticut Hospice, Inc. (1984). *Pastoral Care Policies and Procedures.* Branford, CT.

Cooper, Philip D. (1979). *Health Care Marketing Issues and Trends.* Rockville, MD: Aspen Systems Corporation.

Craven, Joan, and Florence S. Wald. (1975). Hospice Care for Dying Patients. *American Journal of Nursing* 75: 1819.

Cunningham, Robert Jr. (1979). When Enough is Enough. *Hospitals* 53(13): 63-65.

Dailey, Ann A. (1984). *Children's Hospice International Newsletter* (Winter): 1-8.

Department of Health and Human Services, Health Care Financing Administration. (1982). Medicare Program: Comprehensive Outpatient Rehabilitation Facility Services; Final Rule. *Federal Register*. December 15.

_____. (1983). Conditions of Participation for Hospice Benefits under Medicare. *Federal Register*. December 16.

_____. (1983). Medicare Hospice Survey Report--General Provisions.

_____. (1984). Publication No.: HCFA 02154.

Donovan, Judy A. (1984). Team Nurse and Social Worker--Avoiding Role Conflict. *The American Journal of Hospice Care* 1(1):21-23.

Dooley, Jeanne. (1982). The Corruption of Hospice. *Public Welfare* (Spring): 35-41.

Dressler, D. M. (1978). Becoming an Administrator: The Vicissitudes of Middle Management in Mental Health Organizations. *American Journal of Psychiatry* 135 (3): 357-360.

Drucker, P. F. (1974). *Management: Tasks, Responsibilities and Practices.* New York: Harper and Row.

Dunphy, J. Engelbert. (1979). Rising Above Suffering and Death. *Bulletin of the American College of Surgeons* 64 (4): 10-11.

Fello, Maryanne. (1984). Interview with author. Forbes Hospice, July.

Foster, Zelda. (1979). Standards for Hospice Care: Assumptions and Principles. *Health and Social Work* 4(1): 118-128.

Foy, Virginia L. *(1984).* Workshop on "Arts-In-Hospice" at the National Hospice Organization Annual Meeting, Hartford, CT, November.

Frank B. Hall Consulting Company. (1983). *Hospice Reimbursement Survey.* Hawthorne, NY.

Freud, Sigmund. (1907/1959). *Mourning and Melancholia: Collected Papers.* Vol. 4. New York: Basic Books.

Frickey, Charles L. (1984). Reflections on Rural Hospice Care. *The American Journal of Hospice Care.* 1(1): 6-7.

Galinsky, Ronald C. (1982). Staff Stress and Career Burnout. Chapter in *Care of the Terminally Ill Manual: Guide to Professional Training.* Published jointly by Riverside Hospice, Boonton, NJ, and the Office of Consumer Health Education, Department of Community Environment and Medicine, Rutgers Medical School, Piscataway, NJ.

Gilmore, N. J., R. Beaulier, M. Steben, and M. Laverdiere. (1983). AIDS: Acquired Immunodeficiency Syndrome. *Canadian Medical Association Journal* 128(6): 1281-1284.

Glaser, Barney G., and Anselm L. Strauss. (1965). *Awareness of Dying.* Chicago: Aldine.

Gold, Margaret. (1983). *Life Support: What Families Say About Hospital, Hospice and Home Care for the Fatally Ill.* Mount Vernon, NY: Consumers Union Foundation, Inc. Institute for Consumer Policy Research.

Goldenberg, Ira S. (1979). Hospice: To Humanize Dying. *Bulletin of the American College of Surgeons* 64(4): 6-9.

Goldsmith, Seth B. (1981). *Health Care Management: A Contemporary Perspective.* Rockville, MD: Aspen Systems Corporation.

Graham, Nancy O., ed. (1982). *Quality Assurance In Hospitals.* Rockville, MD: Aspen Systems Corporation.

Guthrie, Dorothea. (1979). Dr. Kubler-Ross: A Positive Acceptance of Death. *Bulletin of the American College of Surgeons* 64(4): 12-13.

Hadlock, Daniel. (1980). President's Message. NHO Membership Newsletter, McLean, VA.

Halper, Thomas. (1979). On Death, Dying and Terminality: Today, Yesterday and Tomorrow. *Journal of Health Politics, Policy and Law* 4(1): 11-29.

Hamilton, Michael, and Helen Reid. (1980). *A Hospice Handbook--A New Way To Care For The Dying.* Grand Rapids, MI: William B. Eerdmans Publishing Company.

Health Resources Publishing. (1984). *Hospice Letter.* 6(6): entire issue.

Healy, William. (1980). Hospice. What Is It? *American Health Care Association Journal* (July): 51-56.

Hendin, David. (1973). *Death as A Fact of Life.* New York: W. W. Norton and Co.

Henig, Robin Marantz. (1983). AIDS: A New Disease's Deadly Odyssey. *New York Times Magazine* (Feb. 6): 28-44.

Herzberg, Frederick, Bernard Mausner, and Barbara Block Snyderman. (1959). *The Motivation To Work.* New York: John Wiley and Sons.

International Work Group in Death, Dying, and Bereavement. (1979). Assumptions and Principles Underlying Standards for Terminal Care. *American Journal of Nursing* 79:296-297.

Jemison-Smith, Pearl, and Patricia Hamm. (1983). Infection Control Update! *Critical Care Update* 3:30-31.

Jenkins, Lowell, and Alicia S. Cook. (1981). The Rural Hospice: Integrating Formal and Informal Helping Systems. Paper presented at the Colorado Social Work Conference, Denver, Colorado.

Jivaff, L. (1979). *Home Care and The Quality of Life.* (E. Prichard, ed.) New York: Columbia Press.

Johnson-Hurzeler, Rosemary, Evelyn Barnum, and John Abbott. (1983). Hospice: The Beginning Or The End? The Impact of TEFRA on Hospice Care In The United States. *University of Bridgeport Law Review* 5(1): 69-105.

Joint Commission on Accreditation of Hospitals. (1983). *Hospice Standards Manual.* Chicago.

_____. (1983). *JCAH Hospice Project.* Chicago.

Jones, Bud. (National Ronald McDonald House Coordinator). (1985). Telephone interview, October 4th.

Kadner, Dennis L., and Eli S. Feldman. (1980). Hospice as Part of the Care Continuum in a Comprehensive Geriatric Center. *The Journal of Long-Term Care Administration* 8:43-49.

Kastenbaum, Robert J. (1977). *Death, Society, and Human Experience.* St. Louis: C.V. Mosby.

Kastenbaum, R., and R. Aisenberg. (1972). *The Psychology of Death.* New York: Springer.

Kelly, Orville. (1985). Patient's Children Have Special Needs. Prepared by Springfield, MO chapter of Make Today Count, Inc., from *Make Today Count* and *Until Tomorrow Comes.*

Kotler, Philip. (1975). *Marketing for Non-Profit Organizations.* Englewood Cliffs, NJ: Prentice-Hall.

_____. (1980). *Marketing Management: Analysis, Planning and Control.* Englewood Cliffs, NJ: Prentice-Hall.

Kubler-Ross, Elisabeth. (1969). *On Death and Dying.* New York: Macmillan.

_____. (1974). *Questions and Answers on Death and Dying.* New York: Macmillan.

_____. 1975). *Death: The Final Stage of Growth.* Englewood Cliffs, NJ: Prentice-Hall.

Levey, Samuel, and Paul N. Loomba. (1973). *Health Care Administration.* Philadelphia: J.B. Lippincott Company.

Liebler, Joan Gratto, Ruth Ellen Levine, and Hyman Leo Dervitz. (1984). *Management Principles for Health Professionals.* Rockville, MD: Aspen Systems Corporation.

Lorenz, Lois. (1980). The Hospice Volunteer, Unique Among Volunteers. *Hospice Forum* 1(3):1-2.

McCann, Barbara A. (1983). Hospice Care: A Challenge and an Opportunity for Discharge Planners. *American Hospital Association Discharge Planning Update* (Fall): 8.

_____. (1984). Lecture given at Governor's Conference on an Alternative Health Delivery System. Hershey, PA.

McCool, Barbara, and Montague Brown. (1977). *The Management Response: Conceptual, Technical and Human Skills of Health Administration.* Philadelphia: W.B. Saunders Company.

McGregor, Douglas. (1960). *The Human Side of Enterprise.* New York: McGraw-Hill.

McNulty, Elizabeth Gilman, and Robert A. Holderby. (1983). *Hospice: A Caring Challenge.* Springfield, IL: Charles C. Thomas.

Magno, Josefina B., M.D. (Executive Director of NHO). (1981). Letter To Membership. August 18th.

Maslow, Abraham. (1954). *Motivation and Personality.* New York: Harper and Row.

Mayers, Marlene G., Ronald B. Norby, and Annita B. Watson. (1977). *Quality Assurance for Patient Care.* New York: Appleton-Century-Crofts.

Menapace, Nancy. (1982). *Proposal for Bereavement Program.* Hospice of Pennsylvania, Inc. Typescript.

Miccio, Betty Lou. (1984). A Practical Approach To Quality Assurance for Hospice. *The American Journal of Hospice Care* 1(3): 14-15.

Milch, Robert, M.D. (1984). Quoted in article, Hospice Care Turns Attention to Children. *USA Today* (October 31):section D, 5-6.

Miller, Dulcy B. (1982). *Long Term Care Administrator's Desk Manual.* New York: Panel Publishers, Inc.

Miller, James D. (Chief Executive Officer, Hospice Foundation, Hospice of Pa., Inc.). (1984). Interview with author, August.

Moran, Libby. (1985). The Most Difficult Person I've Ever Worked with--Dr. Cornwall was Obsessed with A.I.D.S. *Nursing Life* 1:30-31.

Mount, Balfour M. (1974). Death--A Fact of Life? *Crux* 11(3): 6.

_____. (1984). Hospice Expert Sees Doctors' Participation as Key to Programs. *Outreach* 5(5): 5.

Mundinger, Mary O'Neil. (1983). *Home Care Controversy: Too Little, Too Late, Too Costly.* Rockville, MD: Aspen Systems Corporation.

Munley, Anne. (1983). *The Hospice Alternative.* New York: Basic Books.

Munley, Anne, Cynthia S. Powers, and John B. Williamson. (1982). Humanizing Nursing Home Environments: The Relevance of Hospice Principles. *International Journal on Aging and Human Development* 15(4):263-283.

National Association of Social Work. New York Chapter. (1981). *Proposed Policy Statement: Hospice Care.* New York.

National Hospice Organization. (1982). *Standards of a Hospice Program of Care.* Arlington, VA.

_____. (1984). *Hospice News.* 2(5):1.

_____. (1984). *Hospice News.* 2(7):6.

_____. (1984). New Study Shows Hospice Improves Hospital Care. *Hospice News.* 2(5):4.

_____. (1984). *State Hospice Connection.* Arlington, VA.

Noyes, Russell, Jr., and John Clancy. (1977). The Dying Role: Its Relevance To Improved Patient Care. *Psychiatry* 40:41-47.

Ouchi, William. (1981). *Theory Z: How American Business Can Meet The Japanese Challenge.* Reading, MA: Addison-Wesley.

Parkes, Colin M. (1972). *Bereavement.* New York: International Universities Press.

Pelletier, K. (1977). *Mind As Healer, Mind As Slayer.* New York: Dell.

Pennsylvania Hospice Network. (1984). Handout, April 27th.

Popkin, Barbara. (1983). Nursing Ground Rounds--Caring for the AIDS Patient--Fearlessly *Nursing 83* 13(9): 50-55.

Pryga, Ellen A., and Henry J. Bachofer. (1983). *Hospice Care Under Medicare: A Working Paper.* Chicago: American Hospital Association, Office of Public Policy Analysis.

Reiss, Kay. (1982). *Hospice Care: A Federal Role?* Congressional Research Service, Library of Congress, Report No. 82-49 EPW, March 22nd.

Rich, Spencer. (1984). 2 Hospice Pioneers Starting a Business. *The Federal Report, The Washington Post,* February 22nd.

Rodek, Christine F., and Susan Jacob. (1983). Perspectives on Hospice. *Cancer Nursing* 6(3): 183.

Roche, K.A. (1980). *Sharing the Experience of Death: A Manual of Family Care.*

Rosen, Harry M., and William Feigin. (1983). Quality Assurance and Data Feedback. *Health Care Management Review* 8(1): 67-74.

Ross, Diane M. (1978). Medicine and Medicaid Hospice Projects. *Journal of American Insurance* 54(2): 209.

Rossman, Parker. (1979). *Hospice.* New York: Fawcett Columbine.

Rubright, Robert, and Dan MacDonald. (1981). *Marketing Health and Human Services.* Rockville, MD: Aspen Systems Corporation.

Rush, Harold M. (1969). *Behavioral Science Concepts and Management Application.* New York: The Conference Board, Inc.

Salloday, Susan A. (1984). Role Playing for Hospice Caregivers. *The American Journal of Hospice Care* 1(2): 26.

Schoenberg, B., and A. C. Carr. (1972). *Psychosocial Aspects of Terminal Care.* New York: Columbia University Press.

Seguine, Arlene. (1983). Relating Medicine To Education--A Curriculum Outline. In *Hospice U.S.A.,* edited by Austin H. Kutscher, et al. New York: Columbia University Press.

Sewell, Marshall, Jr. (1984a). Hospice Medicare Applications Continue to Lag. *Hospice Letter* 6(12).

_____. (1984b). Leader Forms For Profit Hospice Company. *Hospice Letter* 5(12).

Shubin, S. (1978). The Professional Hazard You Face in Nursing. *Nursing* 8(7):25.

Somers, Ann. (1972). The Nation's Health: Issues for the Future. *The Annuals* 399:166-174.

SoRelle, Ruth. (1985). Nursing Care for the AIDS Patient Requires Multiple Skills, Strict Adherence to Procedure. *Oncology Times* 7(2): 1-19.

Spiegel, Allen D. (1983). *Home Healthcare.* Owings Mills, MD: National Health Publishing.

Starr, Paul. (1982). *The Social Transformation of American Medicine.* New York: Basic Books.

Stewart, Sally Ann. (1984). Hospice Care Turns Attention to Children. *USA Today* (October 31):section D, 5-6.

Stoddard, Sandal. (1978). *The Hospice Movement.* Briarcliff Manor, NY: Stein and Day.

Thoreen, Peter W. (1981). *Death, Dying and Terminal Care: Issues Faced By The Long-Term Care Facility.* Minneapolis, MN: Long-Term Care Committee of the Minnesota Coalition for Terminal Care. Inc.

Torrens, Paul R. (1985). *Hospice Programs and Public Policy.* Chicago: American Hospital Publishing, Inc.

Ufema, Joy. (1984). Personal Concerns of Hospice Movement. *The American Journal of Hospice Care* 1(1):5.

U. S. General Accounting Office. (1979). *Hospice Care--A Growing Concept in the United States.* HRD 79-50, March 6.

Vachon, M. L. S. (1982). Are Your Patients Burning Out? *Canadian Family Physician* 28:1570-1574.

_____. (1983). Staff Stress in Care of the Terminally Ill in *Hospice Care Principles and Practice*, edited by Charles A. Carr and Donna M. Carr. New York: Springer.

Vachon, M. L. S., W. A. Lyall, and S. J. J. Freeman. (1978). Measurement and Management of Stress in Health Professionals Working with Advanced Cancer Patients. *Death Education* 1:365-375.

Van Fleteren, Frederick. (1983). *Explaining Death To Children*. Brochure. Quakertown, PA: Ever-Kare, Inc.

Wald, Florence S., Zelda Foster, and Henry J. Wald. (1980). The Hospice Movement As A Health Care Reform. *Nursing Outlook* 28(3):173-178.

Ward, B. J. (1978). Hospice Home Care Program. *Nursing Outlook* 26 (10): 646-49.

Wehr, Frederick T. (1980). *Toward a Gentler Dying Hospice Care In A General Hospital*. Baltimore: A. S. Abell Foundation.

White, Stephen L. (1981). *Managing Health and Human Service Programs: A Guide for Managers*. New York: The Free Press.

Williamson, John B., Linda Evans, and Anne Munley. (1980). *Aging and Society*. New York: Holt, Rinehart and Winston.

Wilson, Barry P., Raymond W. Blosse, Jon L. Tucker, and Kristin K. Spector. (1983). *Hospice Care: Perspectives On A Blue Cross Plan's Community Pilot Program*. Washington, DC: Blue Cross/Blue Shield Association.

Worby, Cyril M., Karen S. Blackman, and John Schneider. (1978). Hospice Care: Current Status and Future Prospects. *Patient Counseling and Health Education* 6(4):61-63.

Zangwill, Willard I. (1976). *Success with People--The Theory Z Approach to Mutual Achievement*. Homewood, IL: Dow-Jones-Irwin.

Zimmerman, Jack M. (1981). *Hospice: Complete Care For The Terminally Ill*. Baltimore-Munich: Urban and Schwarzenberg.

For Further Reading

Ames, Richard P., David Mineau, and Kathy Petrushevich. (1979). Mercy Hospice: A Hospital-based Program. *Hospital Progress* 4 (March): 63-67.

Armado, Anthony, Beatrice A. Cronk, and Rich Mileo. (1979). Cost of Terminal Care: Home Hospice vs. Hospital. *Nursing Outlook* 27 (August): 522-526.

Baird, S. B. (1980). Nursing Roles in Continuing Care: Home Care and Hospice. *Seminars in Oncology* 7 (March): 28-38.

Barstow, J. (1980). Stress Variance In Hospice Nursing. *Nursing Outlook* 28 (December): 751-754.

Bean, I. W. (1978). Care of the Patient with Terminal Cancer. *Primary Care* 5 (December): 731-736.

Beszterezey, A. (1977). Staff Stress on a Newly Developed Palliative Care Service: The Psychiatrist's Role. *Canadian Psychiatric Association Journal* 22: 347-353.

Blues, A., et al. (1980). Hospice Care For The Terminally Ill. *Journal of Kentucky Medical Association* 78 (November): 658-661.

Breindel, Charles L. (1979). Should Hospices be Encouraged? *American Health Care Association Journal* (September): 40-44.

Breindel, Charles L., and Russel M. Boyle. (1979). Implementing a Multiphased Hospice Program. *Hospital Progress* 4 (March): 42-45.

Breindel, Charles L., and Timothy O'Hare. (1979). Analyzing the Hospice Market. *Hospital Progress* 60 (October): 52-55.

Brink, G., et al. (1980). Experts Probe Issues Around Hospice Care. *Hospitals* 54 (June 1): 63-67.

Buckingham, R. W. III, et al. (1976). Living with Dying: Use of the Technique of Participant Observation. *Canadian Medical Journal* 115 (December 18): 1211-1215.

Buell, J. S. (1980). Care At St. Christopher's. *Oncology Nursing Forum* 7 (Fall): 20-22.

Butler, R. N. (1979). The Need for Quality Hospice Care. *Quality Review Bulletin* 5 (May): 2-7.

Callan, John P. (1979). The Hospice Movement. *Journal of the American Medical Association* 241 (February 9): 600.

Cassileth, Barrie R. (1980). Hospice--The Rise and Implications of a New Addition to the Health Care Scene. *Health Law Project Library Bulletin* 5 (June): 189-195.

Chamberlain, A. (1980). Hospice: A Gift of Love. *Texas Nursing* 54 (September): 8-10.

Chiriboga, D. A., G. Jenkins, and J. Bailey. (1983). Stress and Coping Among Hospice Nurses: Test of an Analytic Model. *Nursing Research* 32(5): 294-299.

Churchill, L. R. (1979). Interpretations of Dying: Ethical Implications for Patient Care. *Ethics in Science and Medicine* 6: 211-222.

Clarke, D. (1980). Nursing Care At A Hospice. *Nursing Times* 76 (October 9): 1810.

Coale, J. G. (1979). The Hospice In The Health Care Continuum. *Quality Review Bulletin* 5 (May): 22-23.

Cohen, Sidney. (1978). Heroin Versus Morphine for Pain. *Drug Abuse and Alcoholism Newsletter* 7 (October): 1-3.

Corbett, Terry L., and Dorothy M. Hai. (1979). Searching for Euthanatos: The Hospice Alternative. *Hospital Progress* 4 (March): 38-41.

Cowgill, R. (1980). Hospice Care For The Terminally Ill. *Journal of the Medical Association of Georgia* 69 (April): 264-267.

Davidson, Glen W., ed. (1978). *The Hospice: Development and Administration.* Washington, DC: Hemisphere Publishing Corporation.

_____. (1979). Five Models For Hospice Care. *Quality Review Bulletin* 5 (May): 8-9.

Dellabough, Robin. (1980). Four Models of Hospice Care. *Hospital Forum* 23 (Jan. - Feb.): 15.

Dexter, K. L. (1980). Know Your Community Resources. Hospice Care at Home: An Alternative. *Journal of Gerontological Nursing* 6 (July): 410-411.

Dickinson, George E., and Algene A. Pearson. (1979). Differences in Attitudes Toward Terminal Patients Among Selected Medical Specialties of Physicians. *Medical Care* 17 (June): 682-685.

Dobihal, S. V. (1980). Hospice: Enabling A Patient To Die At Home. *American Journal of Nursing* 80 (August): 1448-1451.

Donovan, Helen. (1980). The Hospice Movement, A Unifying Force? *Nursing Forum* 19: 19-25.

DuBois, Paul M. (1980). *The Hospice Way of Death.* New York: Human Services Press.

Eastman, Margaret. (1978). Shattering Myths About Hospice Care. *American Pharmacy* 18 (November): 20-21.

Falardeau, M., et al. (1979). Palliative Care Unit. *Union Medicale du Canada* 108 (December): 1501-1504.

Farr, William C. (1978). Oral Morphine for Control of Pain in Terminal Cancer. *Arizona Medicine* 35 (March): 167-170.

Fath, Gerlad. (1979). Pastoral Care and the Hospice. *Hospital Progress* 4 (March): 73-75.

Fegenberg, Loma, and R. Fulton. (1977). Care of the Dying: A Swedish Perspective. *Omega* 8: 215-227.

Fennell, F. V. (1980). The Need for Hospices. *New Zealand Medical Journal* 92 (August 27): 158-161.

Flexner, John M. (1979). The Hospice Movement in North America--Is It Coming Of Age? *Southern Medical Journal* 72 (March): 248-250.

Friel, M., et al. (1980). Counteracting Burn-Out for the Hospice Care-Giver. *Cancer Nursing* 3 (August): 285-293.

Garfield, C., and G. Jenkins. (1981). Stress and Coping of Volunteer Grief Counselors. *Omega* 12: 1-13.

Gerson, C. K. (1980). Hospice: People-Centered Care. *American Pharmacy* 201 (June): 27-29.

Gever, L. N. (1980). Brompton's Mixture: How It Relieves The Pain Of Terminal Cancer. *Nursing* (Horsham) 10 (May): 57.

Gibson, M. J. (1978). The Hospice--New Concept in Health Care. *Health Care Horizons*: 32-35.

Glover, D. D., et al. (1980). Brompton's Mixture in Alleviating Pain of Terminal Neoplastic Disease; Preliminary Results. *Southern Medical Journal* 73 (March): 278-282.

Goodman, S. (1979). Hospice Fills Need for Care of Terminally Ill Patients. *Pennsylvania Medicine* 82 (December): 27.

Griffen, Bill, and Dan Blazer. (1979). Hospice in North Carolina; Background and Unanswered Questions. *North Carolina Medical Journal* 40 (April): 208-211.

Hackley, John A. (1977). Full Service Hospice Offers Home, Day and Inpatient Care. *Hospitals* 51 (November 1): 26-29.

_____. (1979). Financing and Accrediting Hospices. *Hospital Progress* (March): 51-53.

Hailstone, Patrick. (1979). The Growing Role of the Hospice. *Health Care in Canada* (April): 44-45.

Haver, T., et al. (1980). Hospice: A Concept of Care in Nursing. *Imprint* 27 (February): 30-32, 67-68.

Hinton, John. (1979). Comparison of Places and Policies for Terminal Care. *Lancet* 1 (January 6): 29-32.

Hodges, Louis F. (1979). Third-Party Payment and Treatment of the Dying. *Ethics in Science and Medicine* 6: 223-228.

Holden, Constance. (1976). Hospices: For The Dying, Relief from Pain and Fear. *Science* 193 (July 30): 389-391.

_____. (1980). Supporting Hospice Care. *Science* 207 (January 11): 160-161.

Hollander, Neil, and David Ehrenfried. (1979). Reimbursing Hospice Care: A Blue Cross and Blue Shield Perspective. *Hospital Progress* 4 (March): 54-56.

Iglehart, John K. (1978). Report of National Hospice Organization Meeting. *Hospital Progress* (November): 20-21.

Kassakian, Marie G., et al. (1979). The Cost and Quality of Dying: A Comparison of Home and Hospital. *Nurse Practitioner* 4 (Jan.-Feb.): 18-19.

Keith, Pat M., and Mary R. Castles. (1979). Expected and Observed Behaviors of Nurses and Terminal Patients. *International Journal of Nursing Studies* 16: 21-28.

King, A. P. (1980). The Bedside Nurse in Terminal Care: A Death At Home. *Journal of Practical Nursing* 30 (June): 23, 40.

Klutch, Murray. (1978). Hospices for Terminally Ill Patients--The California Experience. *Western Journal of Medicine* 129 (July): 82-84.

Klutch, Murray, and Donald P. Holmes. (1980). The Hospice in 1980: A Concept Coming of Age. *Socioeconomic Report* 20 (March).

Kohn, Judith. (1976). Hospice Movement Provides Humane Alternative for Terminally Ill Patients. *Modern Healthcare* 6 (September): 26-28.

_____. (1978). Hospice Group Seeks Reimbursement. *Modern Healthcare* 8 (October): 29.

Kohut, Jeraldine Marasco, and Sylvester Kohut. (1984). *Hospice: Caring For The Terminally Ill.* Springfield, IL: Charles C. Thomas.

Kolbe, Richard. (1977). Inside the English Hospice. *Hospitals* 51 (July 1): 65-67.

Krant, Melvin J. (1978). Sounding Board: The Hospice Movement. *New England Journal of Medicine* 299 (September 7): 546-549.

Kutscher, Austin H., Samuel C. Klagsbrun, Richard J. Torpie, Robert DeBellis, Mahlon S. Hale, and Margot Tallmer, eds. (1983). *Hospice U.S.A.* New York: Columbia University Press.

Lack, Sylvia A. (1979). Hospice--A Concept of Care in the Final Stage of Life. *Connecticut Medicine* 43: 367-372.

Lack, Sylvia A., and Robert W. Buckingham, III. (1978). *First American Hospice; Three Years of Home Care.* New Haven, CT: Hospice, Inc.

Lamerton, Richard C. (1979). Cancer Patients Dying At Home. The Last 24 Hours. *Practitioner* 223 (December): 813-817.

Lattanzi, Marcia, and Diane Coffelt. (1979). *Bereavement Care Manual.* Boulder, CO: Boulder County Hospice, Inc.

Lawrence, S. (1978). New Hospice Opens in Nursing Home. *Forum on Medicine* (September): 18-20.

LeGrand, L. E. (1980). Reducing Burnout in the Hospice and the Death Education Movement. *Death Education* 4(1): 61-75.

Lev, E. L. (1980). An Elective Course in Hospice Nursing. *Oncological Nurses Forum* 8 (Winter): 27-30.

Libman, Joan. (1979). The Hospice Movement. *Medical Times* 107 (May): 1d(108)-2d(108).

Luxton, R. W. (1979). The Modern Hospice and Its Challenge to Medicine. *British Medical Journal* (September 8): 583-584.

McIntier, Sr. Teresa Marie. (1979). Hillhaven Hospice: A Free-standing, Family-centered Program. *Hospital Progress* 4 (March): 68-72.

McNairn, N. (1981), Helping The Patient Who Wants To Die At Home. *Nursing* (Horsham) 11 (February): 66.

McPhee, M. S., R. Arcand, and R. N. MacDonald. (1979). Taking the Stigma Out of Hospice Care: Flexible Approaches for the Terminally Ill. *Canadian Medical Association Journal* 120 (May 19): 1284-1288.

Markel, William M., and Virginia B. Sinon. (1978). The Hospice Concept. *CA-- A Cancer Journal for Clinicians* 28 (July-Aug.): 225-237.

Martin, A. (1981). Hospice Nursing. Walking a Fine Line. *Nursing* (Horsham) 11 (February): 128-130.

Martin, M. Caroline, and Gerald R. Brink. (1980). Setting Up an In-Hospital Hospice. *Hospital Forum* 23 (Jan.-Feb.): 12-14.

Matthews, B. (1980). Setting Up Terminal Care Units. *Nursing Times* 76 (September 18), suppl. 22: 97-98.

Melzack, R., J. G. Ofiesh, and B. M. Mount. (1979). The Brompton Mixture: Effects on Pain in Cancer Patients. *Canadian Medical Association Journal* 115 (July 17): 125-129.

Meyer, K. A. (1980). The Hospice Concept Integrated with Existing Community Health Care. *Nursing Administration Quarterly* 4 (Spring): 49-54.

Mikolaitis, S. M. (1978). Choosing the Circumstances of Death. *Forum* 2: 19-23.

Millett, Nina. (1979). Hospice: Challenging Society's Approach to Death. *Health and Social Work* 4 (1): 131-150.

Milner, C. J. (1980). Compassionate Care for the Dying Person. *Health and Social Work* 5 (May): 5-10.

Mohns, Edward Berger. (1979). Management of the Terminal Patient. *Medical Times* 107 (March): 2d(96)-10d(96).

Mood, Darlene W., and Barbara A. Lakin. (1979). Attitudes of Nursing Personnel Towards Death and Dying: I. Linguistic Indicators of Avoidance. *Research in Nursing and Health* 2 (June): 53-60.

Mount, B. M., R. Melzack, and K. J. MacKinnon. (1978). The Management of Intractable Pain in Patients With Advanced Malignant Disease. *Journal of Urology* 120 (December): 720-725.

Munro, S., and B. Mount. (1978). Music Therapy in Palliative Care. *Canadian Medical Association Journal* 119 (November 4): 1029-1034.

Nuttal, D. (1980). Bereavement. *Health Visit* 53 (March): 84-86.

Oster, Martin W., Monique Vizel, and Livia R. Turgeon. (1978). Pain of Terminal Cancer Patients. *Archives of Internal Medicine* 138: 1801-1802.

Osterweis, Marian, and Daphne S. Champagne. (1979). The Hospice Movement: Issues in Development. *American Journal of Public Health* 69 (May): 492-496.

Parkes, C. Murray. (1978). Home or Hospital? Terminal Care As Seen By Surviving Spouses. *Journal of the Royal College of General Practitioners* 28 (January): 19-30.

_____. (1979). Terminal Care: An Evaluation of Inpatient Service at St. Christopher's Hospice. *Postgraduate Medical Journal* 55 (August): 517-527.

_____. (1980). Bereavement Counselling: Does It Work? *British Medical Journal* 281 (July 5): 3-6.

Parks, Patricia. (1979). Evaluation of Hospice Care Is Needed. *Hospitals* 53 (November 16): 68-70.

_____. (1979). Hospice Care for Dying Patients: A Look at the Issues. *Trustee* 32 (October): 29-32.

_____. (1979). Hospice Care: Implications for Hospitals. *Hospitals* 53 (March 16): 58.

_____. (1980). Evaluation of Hospice Care Still Needed. *Hospitals* 54 (November 16): 56, 102.

Patterson, W. Bradford, and Claire Tehan. (1979), Hospice: Why all this interest? *New York State Journal of Medicine* 79: 1913-1915.

Perrollaz, L. E. (1981). Public Knowledge of Hospice Care. *Nursing Outlook* 29 (January): 46-48.

Philpot, T. (1980). St. Joseph's Hospice: Death--A Part of Life. *Nursing Mirror* 151 (August 21): 20-23.

Plant, J. (1977). Finding a Home for Hospice Care in the United States. *Hospitals* 51 (July 1): 53-62.

Potter, John F. (1980). A Challenge for the Hospice Movement. *New England Journal of Medicine* 203 (January 3): 53-55.

Putnam, S. T., et al. (1980). Home as a Place to Die. *American Journal of Nursing* 80 (August): 1451-1453.

Radford, C. (1980). Community Nursing--Terminal Care: Nursing Care to the End. *Nursing Mirror* 150 (January 24): 30-31.

Rakove, R. (1979). Hospice Care: A Planning Perspective. *Quality Review Bulletin* 5(5): 10-12.

Raphael, Beverly. (1978). Mourning and the Prevention of Melancholia. *British Journal of Medical Psychology* 51 (December): 303-310.

Raphael, Beverly, and David Maddison. (1976). The Care of Bereaved Adults. *Modern Trends in Psychosomatic Medicine* 3: 491-506.

Rees, W. Dewi, and Sylvia G. Lutkins. (1967). Mortality of Bereavement. *British Medical Journal* 4 (October 7): 13-16.

Rizzo, Robert F. (1978). Hospice; Comprehensive Terminal Care. *New York State Journal of Medicine* 78 (October): 1902-1910.

Rizzo, Robert F., and Linda Rizzo. (1979). Hospice Program; Laws, Guidelines, Implementation. *New York State Journal of Medicine* 79 (July): 1244-1247.

Rovinski, Christine. (1979), Hospice Nursing: Intensive Caring. *Cancer Nursing* 2 (Jan.-Feb.): 19-26.

Rudner, H. L. (1979). Who Is Best Qualified to Care for the Terminally Ill? *Canadian Medical Association Journal* 121 (November 17): 1348, 1315.

Rundles, R. Wayne. (1978). Principles of Palliation. *Medical Times* 106 (March): 112-116.

Russel, P. S. B. (1979). Analgesia in Terminal Malignant Disease. *British Medical Journal* 1 (June 9): 1561.

Ryder, Claire F., and Diane M. Ross. (1977). Terminal Care--Issues and Alternatives. *Public Health Reports* 92 (Jan.-Feb.): 20-29.

Saunders, B. (1980). The Terminal Care Support Team. *Nursing* (Oxford) (July): 657-659.

Saunders, Cicely. (1976). Care for the Dying. *Patient Care* 3 (June).

_____. (1976). The Last Achievement. *Nursing Times* 72 (August 12): 1247-1249.

_____. (1976). Mental Distress in the Dying. *Nursing Times* 72 (July 29): 1172-1174.

_____. (1976). The Nursing of Patients Dying of Cancer. *Nursing Times* (August 5).

_____. (1978). Hospice Care. *American Journal of Medicine* 65 (November): 726-728.

_____, ed. (1978). *The Management of Terminal Disease*. London: Edward Arnold, Ltd.

Schmale, A. H. (1980). The Dying Patient. *Advances in Psychosomatic Medicine* 10: 99-110.

Slack, P. (1980). The Hospice Comes of Age. *Nursing Times* 76 (June 12): 1034.

Smith, C. A., and P. D. H. Hill. (1978). Grieving Responses, A Comparison After Home or Hospital Care. *New Zealand Medical Journal* 88 (November 22): 393-395.

Spiegel, David, and Irwin D. Yalom. (1978). A Support Group for Dying Patients. *International Journal of Group Psychotherapy* 28 (April): 233-245.

Spillane, Edward J. (1979). An Analysis of Catholic-sponsored Hospices. *Hospital Progress* 4 (March): 46-50.

Stedford, Averil, and Sidney Block. (1979). The Psychiatrist in the Terminal Care Unit. *British Journal of Psychiatry* 135: 1-6.

Sweetser, C. (1979). Integrated Care: The Hospital-Based Hospice. *Quality Review Bulletin* (May): 18-21.

Tehan, Claire B. (1980). Standards for Hospice Address Definition and Quality of Care. *Hospital Forum* 23 (Jan.-Feb.): 16.

Toth, S. B., and A. Toth. (1980). Empathetic Intervention With the Widow. *American Journal of Nursing* 80 (September): 1652-1654.

Turnbull, Alan D., et al. (1979). The Inverse Relationships Between Cost and Survival in the Critically Ill Cancer Patient. *Critical Care Medicine* 7 (January): 20-23.

Turnbull, P. R. (1980). The Relationship of the Surgeon to the Patient with Advanced Malignant Disease. *New Zealand Medical Journal* 92 (November 12): 354-356.

Twycross, Robert G. (1977). Choice of Strong Analgesic in Terminal Cancer: Diamorphine or Morphine? *Pain* 3: 93-104.

Vaile, Ivan R. (1979). Hospice or Rehabilitation Hospital? Alternatives for the Terminally Ill. *Canadian Medical Association Journal* 120 (May 19): 1291-92.

Valentour, Louis F. (1979). Hospice Design Keyed to Program Goals. *Hospitals* 54 (February 16): 140-143.

Vanderpool, Harold Y. (1978). The Ethics of Terminal Care. *Journal of the American Medical Association* 239 (February 27): 850-852.

Vere, D. W. (1980). The Hospital as a Place of Pain. *Journal of Medical Ethics* (September 6): 117-119.

Weiss, Rhoda. (1980). Hospital Employees Educated on Hospice. *Hospital Forum* (January).

West, T. S. (1978). Hospice Care for a Dying Person. *Patient Counseling and Health Education* N1 (2): 65-69.

Westbrook, B. B., Jr. (1980). A Review of the Hospice Concept. *Texas Medicine* 76 (June): 45-46.

Wilkes, E., A. G. O. Crowther, and C. W. K. H. Greaves. (1978). A Different Kind of Day Hospital--for Patients with Preterminal Cancer and Chronic Disease. *British Medical Journal* 2 (October 14): 1053-1056.

Willians, J. H. (1979),. Selecting Staff for Hospice Work. *Nursing Times* 75 (December 6), suppl. 32: 129-130.

_____. (1980). Nutrition: Appetite in the Terminally Ill Patient. *Nursing Times* 76 (May 15): 875-876.

Wills, L. A. M. (1978). Continuity of Care for Patients with Malignant Disease. *Postgraduate Medical Journal* 54 (June): 391-394.

Wilson, D. Montreal. (1978). The Royal Victoria Hospital Palliative Care Service. *Death Education* 2 (Spring/Summer): 3-19.

Winder, Alvin E., and Judith R. Elam. (1978). Therapist for the Cancer Patient's Family: A New Role for the Nurse. *Journal of Psychiatric Nursing* 16 (October): 22-27.

Winstead, D. K., et al. (1980). Hospice Consultation Team: A New Multidisciplinary Model. *General Hospital Psychiatry* 2 (September): 169-176.

Worden, J. W. (1982). *Grief Counseling and Grief Therapy.* New York: Springer Publishing.

Yalom, Irvin D., and Carlos Greaves. (1977). Group Therapy with the Terminally Ill. *American Journal of Psychiatry* 134 (April): 396-400.

Yukna, B. J. (1980). Symptomatic Control of the Terminally Ill: Practical Approaches with 250 Patients. *Maryland State Medical Journal* 29 (June): 59-60.

Zimmerman, J. M. (1979). Experience with a Hospice-Care Program for the Terminally Ill. *Annals of Surgery* 189 (June): 683-690.

Index

About the Author

Alice E. McDonnell received her R.N., B.S.N. and doctorate in public health from Columbia University, having done her research in the field of hospice. She also received a master's degree in public administration from Marywood Graduate School of Arts and Sciences.

Currently, Dr. McDonnell is Director of Professional, Clinical, and Educational Operations, Hospice of Pennsylvania Foundation in Scranton, PA, providing management services to health care facilities and organizations, including Hospice of PA, Inc., Scranton, PA; Heritage Nursing Home, Inc., Athens, PA; and Hemodialysis Patients Association of Northeastern PA, among others. In addition, Dr. McDonnell is Chairperson, Department of Public Administration, Marywood Graduate School of Arts and Sciences. She is likewise Chairperson of the Gerontology Institute, Marywood Graduate School of Arts and Sciences and Graduate School of Social Work.

Dr. McDonnell is a board member and a member of the Standards and Licensure Committee, Pennsylvania Hospice Network. She has also served on various other boards and committees, including Lackawanna Mental Health Association, Lackawanna County unit of the American Cancer Society, Northeastern PA Community Hospital Oncology Program, Telespond Senior Services, Inc., Voluntary Action Center, Lackawanna United Way Panel, Hemodialysis Patients Association, and Sigma Theta Tau (National Honor Society of Nursing). Dr. McDonnell resides in Scranton, PA and is frequently consulted on all aspects of hospice care delivery.